I0475649

The Authorities

Powerful Wisdom from Leaders in the Field

MELANIE R. PALOMARES, M.D., M.S.

Physician Founder of Cancer Prevention Inc.

© 2017 by 10-10-10 Publishing

All rights reserved. No part of this publication may be reproduced or transmitted in any form or by any means, electronic or mechanical, including photocopying, recording, or any other information storage and retrieval system without the written permission of the publisher and author.

Limits of Liability and Disclaimer of Warranty
The author and publisher shall not be liable for your misuse of the enclosed material. This book is strictly for informational and educational purposes only.

Warning – Disclaimer
The purpose of this book is to educate and entertain. The author and/or publisher do not guarantee that anyone following these techniques, suggestions, tips, ideas, or strategies will become successful. The author and/or publisher shall have neither liability nor responsibility to anyone with respect to any loss or damage caused, or alleged to be caused, directly or indirectly by the information contained in this book.

Medical Disclaimer
The medical or health information in this book is provided as an information resource only, and is not to be used or relied on for any diagnostic or treatment purposes. This information is not intended to be patient education, does not create any patient-physician relationship, and should not be used as a substitute for professional diagnosis and treatment.

Published by:
10-10-10 PUBLISHING
MARKHAM, ON
CANADA

Printed in the United States of America.

ISBN:978-1542804097

FOREWORD

Experts are to be admired for their knowledge, but they often remain unrecognized by the general public because they save their information and insights for paying customers and clients. There are many experts in a given field, but their impact is limited to the handful of people with whom they work.

Unlike experts, authorities share their knowledge and expertise far more broadly, so they make a big impact on the world. Authorities become known and admired as leading experts and, as such, typically do very well economically and professionally. Most authorities are also mature enough to know that part of the joy of monetary success is the accompanying moral and spiritual obligation to give back.

Many people want to learn and work with well-respected and generous authorities, but don't always know where to find them. They may be known to their peers, or within a specific community, but have not had the opportunity to reach a wider audience. At one time, they might have submitted a proposal to the For Dummies or Chicken Soup for the Soul series of books, but it's now almost impossible to get accepted as a new author in such branded book series.

It is more than fitting that Raymond Aaron, an internationally known and respected authority in his own right, would be the one to recognize the need for a new venue in which authorities could share their considerable knowledge with readers everywhere. As the only author ever to be included in both of the book series mentioned above, Raymond has had the opportunity to give back and he understands how crucial it is for authorities to have a platform from which to share their expertise.

I have known and worked with Raymond for a number of years and consider him a valued friend and talented coach. He knows how to spot talented and knowledgeable people and he desires to see them prosper. Over the years, success coaching and speaking engagements around the world have made it possible for Raymond to meet many of these talented authorities. He recognizes and relates to their passion and enthusiasm for what they do, as well as their desire to share what they know. He tells me that's why he created this new nonfiction branded book series, The Authorities.

Dr. Nido Qubein
President, High Point University

TABLE OF CONTENTS

ACKNOWLEDGEMENTS

To my parents, Bernabe and Elba Palomares, who inspired me to become a physician and entrepreneur, you shaped me into the person that I am today.

To all my teachers, from grade school to high school, college, medical school, graduate school, and post-graduate training, you shaped me into the professional that I am today. I also want to acknowledge my patients and student interns, who were always my very best teachers.

To Lisa Kalmin and the WorldWorks community, who reminded me that I have a voice and I get to use it to support others beyond the patients that I have physically had the privilege to care for.

To the health coaching community, who validated my long-standing belief that true wellness includes not only a healthy body, but also a healthy mind and healthy finances.

To my award-winning co-authors, who contributed to the construction of this book that addresses all three of these domains of wellness.

To Miriam Cohen for her writing assistance. Thank you for your diligence and patience with me.

To my friends and family who took the time to read my drafts and offered me very helpful feedback, which you can see from the finished product that I took to heart.

To you, the reader, for boldly taking the driver's seat in your earthly journey by seeking to inform yourself about what you can do to live a healthy life. While cancer risk, screening, and prevention are very broad topics, I hope that my chapter provides you with a good starting foundation. I invite you to remain connected with me by registering at my website, www.caprevinc.org.

INTRODUCTION

This book introduces you to *The Authorities* — individuals who have distinguished themselves in life and in business. Authorities make a big impact on the world. Authorities are leaders in their chosen fields. Authorities typically do very well financially, and are evolved enough to know that part of the joy of monetary success is the accompanying social, moral and spiritual obligation to give back.

Authorities are not just outstanding. They are also *known* to be outstanding.

This additional element begins to explain the difference between two strategic business and life concepts — one that seems great, but isn't, and the other that fills in the essential missing gap of the first.

The first concept is "the expert."

What is an expert? The real definition is ...

EXPERT: *a person who knows stuff*

People who have attained a very senior academic degree (like a PhD or an MD) definitely know stuff. People who read voraciously and retain what they read definitely know stuff. Unfortunately, just because you know stuff does not mean that anyone respects the fact that you do. Even though some experts are successful, alas, most are not — because knowing stuff is not enough.

Well, then, what is the missing piece?

What the expert lacks, "the authority" has. The authority both knows stuff and is *known* to know stuff. So, more simply ...

AUTHORITY: *a person who is known as an expert*

The difference is not subtle. The difference is not merely semantic. The difference is enormous.

When it comes to this subject, there are actually three categories in which people fall:

- People who don't know much and are unsuccessful in life and in business. Most people fall in this category.

- People who know stuff, but still don't leave much of a footprint in the world. There are a lot of people like this.

- Experts who are also *known* as experts become authorities and authorities are always wondrously successful. Authorities are able to contribute more to humanity through both their chosen work and their giving back.

This book is about the highest category, *The Authorities* — people who have reached the peak in their field and are known as such.

You will definitely know some of The Authorities in this book, especially since there are some world-famous ones. Our featured author, Melanie. R. Palomares, M.D., M.S, has held a variety of posts in multiple national scientific organizations, including the American Society of Clinical Oncologists (ASCO), the American Society of Preventive Oncology (ASPO), American Association for Cancer Research (AACR) and Southwest Oncology Group (SWOG), and her groundbreaking work has been featured in the such magazines as International Innovation and Family Circle. Her unique multidisciplinary medical training in Internal Medicine, Hematology-Oncology, Epidemiology, and Cancer Genetics, as well as her professional experience as co-founder of the City of Hope High Risk Breast Clinic and, more recently, Physician Founder of Cancer Prevention, Inc., makes her a true authority, both in primary cancer prevention and screening among people with an increased risk for cancer and in secondary cancer prevention and surveillance among cancer survivors. Affectionately known as Dr. Mel, she has her own personal health transformation story, which includes a 20% body weight loss, blood pressure normalization without medications, and a curative surgery for a premelanoma. She is an example of using healthy nutrition, physical activity, and early detection to promote health and prevent disease. Dr. Palomares' chapter is about recognizing what you can and cannot control, and her wise words will empower you to mitigate your own chances of developing cancer.

Read each chapter carefully to learn and to see the business potential that may be possible between yourself and each one of *The Authorities*. You may well be able to become their client or, possibly, do business with them in other ways.

They are *The Authorities*. Learn from them. Connect with them. Let them uplift you. Learning from them and working with them is the secret ingredient for success which may well allow you to rise to the level of Authority soon.

To be considered for inclusion in a subsequent edition of *The Authorities*, register to attend a future event at www.aaron.com/events where you will be interviewed and considered.

The Greatest Weapon Against Cancer Is Knowledge

Every Cancer Is Different. Learn About Your Risk And Ways to Reduce It

MELANIE R. PALOMARES, M.D., M.S.

C ancer afflicts millions of people and takes hundreds of thousands of lives each year. In 2012, the World Health Organization (WHO) reported 14 million new cancer diagnoses and 8.2 million deaths— and that number is projected to rise in the coming years.[1] Statistics suggest that about 39 percent of men and women will be diagnosed with this disease at some point during their lifetime.[2] The good news is that, today, early

---

1 World Health Organization Staff, "WHO | Cancer." World Health Organization, 2015. Web. http://www.who.int/mediacentre/factsheets/fs297/en/

2 National Cancer Institute Staff, "SEER Stat Fact Sheets: Cancer of Any Site." National Cancer Institute, 2013. Web. https://seer.cancer.gov/statfacts/html/all.html

detection and specialized treatment for different types of cancer can make all the difference.

Cancer used to be the disease that no one talked about—and, unfortunately, that meant that people at risk didn't even know about their family's medical history. Even today, there's a stigma surrounding cancer patients. In an article for *Cancer World*, the principal periodical of the European School of Oncology, Associate Editor Anna Wagstaff gives a harrowing report of the way societies around the world view cancer:

"Fears that the disease may be infectious can result in people being shunned by friends and neighbours (sic) and excluded from the community. Fears that it is hereditary can ruin the marriage chances of those with a mother or father known to have had cancer. Whole families can find themselves impacted, which can then put intolerable strains on relationships, leaving people with cancer even more isolated."[3]

The good news is that we are far more educated on the matter than we used to be. Today we have a wealth of information available via social media and the internet. The challenge is the quality of information available from such sources, which are not always subject to medical peer review. This has led to more awareness, and there have been more discoveries about lifestyle and environmental risk factors, which may be modified to improve cancer risk.

Studies have shown that the more accurate information one has, the better chance one has to maintain their health. In general, you are far more likely to survive a bout with cancer if you catch it at an early stage. For instance, Mayo Clinic reports the survival rate for colorectal cancer is 90% if it is caught early, although it is the second deadliest cancer in the United States, when all stages

---

3 World Health Organization Staff, "WHO | Cancer." World Health Organization, 2015. Web. http://www. Anna Wagstaff, "Stigma: Breaking the Vicious Cycle." Cancer World, 2013. Web. http://www.cancerworld. org/Articles/Issues/55/July-August-2013/Patient-Voice/602/Stigma-breaking-the-vicious-cycle.html

are considered.[4]

This information may motivate you to pursue cancer screenings, but you should know that those come with their own set of risks. For one thing, screening tests are not 100% reliable. Even when they are conducted by medical professionals you know and trust, the possibility of a false-positive or false-negative result exists. Beyond that, some testing procedures come with their own immediate hazards. Colonoscopies, for example, carry some risk of damaging the lining of the colon.[5] Therefore, it is important to pursue to proper type and frequency of screening for your level of cancer risk.

By far, the best defenses against cancer are prevention and proactivity. The National Cancer Institute estimates that as many as 50-75% of cancer fatalities in the United States are caused by negative lifestyle choices, like smoking, lack of exercise, or poor diet.[6] Just by living a healthy lifestyle, you can reduce your chances of contracting cancer dramatically.

That said, it is most important to know how prone you are to the disease. If the disease runs in your family, or if you think that you may have had an exposure that may increase your risk of developing cancer (examples of such risk factors are discussed throughout this chapter), you need not feel helpless. Your first step is to talk with an oncologist or a general physician with specific training and experience in understanding cancer risk factors to perform an accurate risk assessment. From there, you can obtain personalized cancer screening recommendations tailored to your level of risk. You can also learn about a variety of different precautions that you can take to minimize

---

4 Sharon Theimer, "Mayo Clinic Expert Shares Five Things to Know About Colorectal Cancer." Mayo Clinic News Network, 2016. Web. http://newsnetwork.mayoclinic.org/discussion/mayo-clinic-expert-shares-5-things-to-know-about-colorectal-cancer/

5 National Cancer Institute, "Cancer Screening Overview." National Cancer Institute, 2016. Web. https://www.cancer.gov/about-cancer/screening/patient-screening-overview-pdq

6 National Cancer Institute, NIH, DHHS. Cancer Trends Progress Report – 2011/2012 Update. Bethesda; 2012.

your chances of developing any form of cancer. It all comes down to having a keen knowledge of your personal history and knowing exactly what your body needs at any given time in your life, based on your age and occurrences in your life.

EVALUATING YOUR RISKS

When evaluating and minimizing your risk of developing cancer, it is important to note that one size does not fit all. Each form of cancer comes with a specific and distinct set of risk factors, variables that make you more or less susceptible to cancer development. In general, risk factors for cancer can be filed under two different classifications: genetic and environmental.

Genetic Risk Factors Are Inborn

Those with family histories of cancer, or those who inherit mutated genes from their parents, often have a relatively high chance of developing cancer. By nature, genetic risks are immutable and unalterable; we cannot, after all, change the way we were born. However, it is still important to recognize how your genes affect your chances of developing cancer, so that you may take appropriate preventive measures.

Environmental Risk Factors Are a Product of Nurture

These risk factors revolve around the characteristics of your living area, such as the climate (eg. sun exposure), the quality of the air you breathe, and the food you consume. Unlike genetic factors, environmental factors are, to some extent, subject to change. However, these changes may or may not be within your control, depending on what your living options are and whether you can afford to move.

In general, while there are many types and subtypes of cancer, all associated with different risk factors, screening, treatment, and prevention, in this chapter I will focus on the four most common cancers in the U.S.: breast and gynecologic cancers, colon cancer, lung cancer, and prostate cancer. These "Big Four" account for over 50% of all the cancers that occur in Americans.

BREAST AND GYNECOLOGIC CANCERS

From birth, sex hormones play an instrumental role in your body's growth, maturity and fertility. After you mature, your reproductive health is largely dependent on how well your body maintains the balance between estrogens and androgens. The enzyme aromatase plays a particularly vital part in a woman's reproductive health, breaking down larger hormones in the breasts and ovaries. This is important to note because breast cancer, like most gynecologic cancers, is hormone-driven.

The most important factors in determining breast cancer risk are gender and age. Since breast cancer growth is facilitated by the presence of female hormones, it serves to reason that the illness predominately affects women (but not only women). It also follows that breast cancer is most likely to develop post-maturity, when the body's hormonal activity reaches its peak. This is also the case for most ovarian and uterine cancers. On the other hand, cervical cancer is more likely to occur in young women, particularly those with more sexual activity, though the availability of human papilloma virus (HPV) vaccines will likely change the epidemiology of that disease as they become more commonly used for cancer prevention in girls and young women.

With breast and gynecologic cancers, despite popular belief, the role of inheritance is relatively minor. Although a family history of breast and/or ovarian cancer does make it more likely that you will develop one of these diseases, studies show that less than 15-20% of diagnosed breast cancer patients in America have immediate relatives with the same affliction,[7] and only about 5-10% have a strong family history of breast and/or ovarian cancer associated with a high cancer susceptibility genetic mutation. The most well-known examples are inherited mutations in the BRCA1 or BRCA2 genes, which are associated with the Hereditary Breast and Ovarian Cancer (HBOC) syndrome. Yet other cancer susceptibility genetic mutations, specifically mutations the DNA mismatch repair genes, are associated with a high risk of uterine and ovarian cancer with colon cancer, rather than breast cancer, in an entirely different inheritable entity called Lynch syndrome. In addition, there are gene mutations that carry only an intermediate elevation in risk for developing breast cancer, such as inherited mutations in a gene called PTEN, which are also associated with uterine cancer, thyroid cancer, and colon polyps as part of a less common familial entity called Cowden's syndrome. While there are even a few more familial syndromes that have been described to be associated with breast and/or gynecologic cancer, cervical cancer appears to be related to HPV infection as an environmental risk, with little to no relation to inheritance.

In addition to family history, you should also look into your personal history; breast cancer is more likely to happen in women who had their first period before age 12, as well as those who went through menopause relatively late.[8] The standard use of mammograms for breast cancer screening since the 1980s has shifted this disease to one that is more often caught early, except in younger women who may not have started regular screening yet. Two points

---

7 breastcancer.org Staff, "U.S. Breast Cancer Statistics." breastcancer.org, 2016. Web. http://www.breastcancer.org/symptoms/understand_bc/statistics
8 Mayo Clinic Staff, "Symptoms and Causes – Breast Cancer." Mayo Clinic, 2016. Web. http://www.mayoclinic.org/diseases-conditions/breast-cancer/symptoms-causes/dxc-20207918

follow from this trend: 1) women who have had findings of changes that occur prior to the development of a full cancer have an opportunity for medical prevention, and 2) it is particularly important to understand a woman's cancer risk in order to adjust screening recommendations to given high-risk women the same opportunity for early detection.

Lastly, diet and physical activity appear to play an important role in the development of these cancers. Obesity has been particularly associated with breast and uterine cancer. In addition, excessive alcohol use has been linked to breast cancer risk, particularly in premenopausal women.

COLORECTAL CANCERS

Colorectal cancers originate in the colon and rectum. The term "colorectal cancer" refers the most common of the cancers that develop within the human digestive tract. Colorectal cancers share a variety of causes and risk factors. One of them is chronic inflammation, as is seen in individuals with a history of the chronic inflammatory bowel diseases (IBD), Crohn's Disease or Ulcerative Colitis. Chronic inflammation can lead to the development of dysplasia, abnormally structured cells in the colon. Dysplastic cells often contain somatic, or non-inherited genetic mutations that are acquired after birth, which have the potential to develop into cancer cells over time.

Also, like breast and ovarian cancers, colorectal cancers have a familial component. In fact, there are some hereditary conditions that increase their carriers' propensity towards colorectal cancer. One such condition is Lynch syndrome, which was mentioned in the previous section, because of its association with uterine and ovarian cancers as well. Another syndrome is called familial adenomatous polyposis (FAP), an inherited condition that causes multiple polyps to grow in the patient's large intestine.[9] There are additional familial syndromes that have been described to be associated with colorectal cancers. These, as well as more detail about other cancer genetics syndromes, may be found at my website, www.caprevinc.org.

Diet is also thought to play a role in colon cancer, with certain elements, such as adequate folate and fiber intake, appearing to take an important role in minimizing risk.[10] Diets that include lots of vegetables, fruits, and whole grains have also been linked with a decreased risk of colon cancer. Dietary fat has been linked to a higher risk of colon cancer, as well as tobacco and alcohol use. The American Institute for Cancer Risk (AICR) estimates that 45% of colon cancers are preventable through diet, staying a healthy weight, and being physically active.[11]

LUNG CANCER

In general, lifestyle and environmental factors play the largest role in the development of lung cancer. This is an important point, in that lung cancer is the most common cause of cancer death in the United States, yet its risk factors are largely modifiable. Thus, it is important to understand these risks so that you can make the best choices for yourself and your family.

While tobacco use is the most well known risk factor, an additional major contributing factor is the exposure to secondhand smoke, or smoke expelled from used cigarettes and tobacco pipes. The American Cancer Society has

9 Al-Sukhni W, Aronson M, Gallinger S. "Hereditary colorectal cancer syndromes: familial adenomatous polyposis and lynch syndrome." Surg Clin North Am. 2008 Aug;88(4):819-44, vii. doi: 10.1016/j.suc.2008.04.012.

10 Giovannucci E, Willett WC. "Dietary factors and risk of colon cancer." Ann Med. 1994 Dec;26(6):443-52.

11 http://www.aicr.org/press/press-releases/preventing-colon-cancer-6-steps.html?referrer=https://www.google.com/

shown that secondhand smoke is even more toxic and carcinogenic than the vapor taken in by smokers themselves.[12] Because of this, the risk of lung cancer is relatively high for those who live or work around chronic smokers. Smoking and other tobacco use, such as chewing tobacco, also increases the risk for aerodigestive cancers, such as cancers of the oral cavity, throat, esophagus, and stomach. And because tobacco products can be excreted in the urine, tobacco use is also associated with kidney and bladder cancer.

Another large contributing factor to lung cancer is radon poisoning. Radon is a colorless, odorless substance that spawns from the natural decay of uranium in soil. Commonly, homes, particularly those in suburban or rural areas, can build up large quantities of radon over time as it rises up from the soil and seeps through cracks and flaws in the foundation. This is more common than you might think; in fact, it's responsible for roughly 21,000 lung cancer deaths each year, making it the second largest contributor to lung cancer behind tobacco.[13]

Asbestos is another major environmental factor associated with lung cancer. Asbestos poisoning is associated with a specific kind of lung cancer called mesothelioma. Since the 1980s, several laws have been passed in this country to restrict the availability and usage of asbestos in architecture. In spite of this, we still see a steady number of new mesothelioma diagnoses each year—about 3,000 annually, as estimated by the Mesothelioma Center.[14]

---

12 American Cancer Society, "Health Risks of Secondhand Smoke." ACS, 2015. Web. http://www.cancer.org/cancer/cancercauses/tobaccocancer/secondhand-smoke

13 Janet McCabe, "For peace of mind, add 'test for radon' to your 2016 to-do list." EPA Connect, 2016. Web.https://blog.epa.gov/blog/2016/01/test-for-radon/

14 The Mesothelioma Center, "Mesothelioma - Overview of Malignant Mesothelioma Cancer." asbestos.org, 2016. Web. https://www.asbestos.com/mesothelioma/

PROSTATE CANCER

Prostate cancer is the most common cancer occurring in American men, aside from skin cancer.[15] In 2016 alone, 26,120 American men were reported to have died from this affliction. In fact, one in seven men will be diagnosed with prostate cancer in their lifetime. Like breast and gynecologic cancers, prostate cancer is largely influenced by hormones; the difference, of course, is that it feeds off of androgens, male hormones, rather than estrogens.

Age is also a risk factor. Prostate cancer is seldom diagnosed in men younger than 40, and roughly 60% of cases are diagnosed in men at least 65 years of age.[16] Heredity and genes also play a role in prostate cancer development, although no highly penetrant cancer susceptibility genes have been described to date, unlike with breast, gynecologic, and colorectal cancers. Nevertheless, men who are closely related to prostate cancer patients are twice as likely to develop it themselves. The risk heightens even further if a man has more than one affected relative.

CANCER SCREENING

Cancer screening methods range from physical exam or self-exam to blood tests and specialized x-rays, such as mammograms, or procedures, such as colonoscopies. These methods are recommended to be performed at different frequencies depending upon age, family history, and other risk factors.

Concerns about false positive results, which can lead to unnecessary tests

---

15 Rebecca L. Siegel, Kimberly D. Miller and Ahmedin Jemal, "Cancer Statistics, 2016." CA: A Cancer Journal for Clinicians, 2016. Web. http://onlinelibrary.wiley.com/doi/10.3322/caac.21332/full

16 Prostate Cancer Foundation, "Prostate Cancer FAQs." Web. http://www.pcf.org/site/c.leJRIROrEpH/b.5800851/k.645A/Prostate_Cancer_FAQs.htm

and patient anxiety, as well as to overdiagnosis and overtreatment, has led to widespread controversy regarding different screening techniques. In addition, due to concerns about health care costs, cancer screening policies differ from country to country. This is why different guidelines are often offered by different medical organizations, which unfortunately leads to confusion for both consumers and health care professionals.

It is for this reason that I highly recommend seeking the advice of a physician with specific training and experience in understanding cancer risk factors to perform an accurate risk assessment. From there, you can obtain personalized recommendations specified to your risk level. Resources for determining your general category of cancer risk and, if appropriate, how to find a referral to a qualified health care professional near you can be found at my website, www. caprevinc.org. Webinars on this topic are in development and will be available at that site as well.

REDUCING YOUR RISK

While cancer screening can help with early detection of cancer, which does improve outcomes with cancer treatment, as mentioned earlier in this chapter, it is important to remember that you have the power to help mitigate your chances of developing cancer in the first place (or getting it again, if you are a cancer survivor). Fighting the disease is a matter of recognizing what you can and cannot control, and focusing on what you can control. Your personal choices on a day-to-day basis can make a huge difference in your personal war against cancer, and you cannot go into battle without knowing what the consequences of those choices are.

LIFESTYLE INTERVENTIONS

A balanced, careful diet is key to fighting cancer. The influence of your food intake on your cancer risk cannot be overstated. Some foods actually have the potential to increase your risk of developing cancer, so it's vital to know what to eat, what to abstain from, and what to limit.

Diet: Plant-Based Foods

When it comes to prevention of and survivorship with cancer, fruits, vegetables and whole grains are the most desirable foods you can eat. Cancer.net educates patients about the link between excessive body fat and the development of several types of cancer, including the aforementioned colorectal cancer.[17] As such, your best bet is to eat foods that are low in fat and high in fiber. Plant-based food groups (vegetables, fruits, nuts, whole grains and legumes) all fit the bill. Fiber-rich foods in particular will help you along the way. Fiber is the broom of the digestive system, sweeping your intestines clean and keeping your digestive processes running at regular intervals. Because of this, fiber helps flush carcinogenic compounds out of your body, thus preventing cancer from growing.

Diet: Animal Products

While a plant-based diet is wholly important to cancer prevention, this does not mean you have to swear off meat and dairy altogether. You should, however, place significant limits on how much animal-based food you take in. Most people, especially Americans, consume far more meat than they should.

---

17 Cancer.net Editorial Board, "Obesity, Weight and Cancer Risk." Cancer.net, 2016. Web. http://www.cancer.net/navigating-cancer-care/prevention-and-healthy-living/obesity-and-cancer/obesity-weight-and-cancer-risk

In general, meat should not constitute more than a small fraction of the calories you take in per day. It's also important to recognize that some meats are better than others. Poultry and fish, for instance, are leaner and healthier alternatives to beef and pork. It's also a good idea to stay away from processed meats, like hot dogs and salami.

Physical Activity

Get moving! Exercise, particularly aerobic exercise, is an integral part of weight management, and by extension, cancer prevention. It is possible to reduce your risk for colorectal and breast cancer in particular with a regular exercise regimen. The AICR recommends sustained physical activity for at least 30 minutes a day.[18]

In addition to avoidance of obesity, which has been linked to an increasing number of different cancer types,[19] there are other benefits provided by regular exercise. For one thing, it keeps your metabolism running quickly and efficiently, which in turn will keep your weight at a healthy level. It also serves to strengthen your immune system, which plays an integral role in your body's defenses against cancer. Finally, regular exercise helps regulate your hormone levels which, as mentioned before, play a key role in the development of gynecologic cancers.

---

18 American Institute for Cancer Research, "Physical Activity Recommended for Preventing Cancer." AICR, 2016. Web. http://www.aicr.org/reduce-your-cancer-risk/recommendations-for-cancer-prevention/recommendations_02_activity.html

19 Béatrice Lauby-Secretan, Ph.D., Chiara Scoccianti, Ph.D., Dana Loomis, Ph.D., Yann Grosse, Ph.D., Franca Bianchini, Ph.D., and Kurt Straif, M.P.H., M.D., Ph.D., for the International Agency for Research on Cancer Handbook Working Group. Body Fatness and Cancer — Viewpoint of the IARC Working Group. N Engl J Med 2016; 375:794-798, August 25, 2016.

Stress Management

Chronic stress can affect body system functioning, particularly the immune system, and a weak immune system makes the body a more hospitable environment for cancer cells to grow. Stress also leads to release of a hormone called cortisol, which leads to truncal obesity, thereby leading to an increased risk of obesity-related cancers. Cortisol, along with other stress-related chemicals called catecholamines, has also been shown to directly facilitate cancer growth. Yet other stress hormones can inhibit a process called anoikis, which normally kills diseased cells and prevents them from spreading. Finally, chronic stress leads to increased production of growth factors that promote inflammation and new blood supply, which could potentially feed a developing cancer, as well as provide an environment for invasion and metastasis, or spread.[20]

While it is not realistic to avoid all sources of stress in our lives, it is possible to manage our relationship to external stressors. Mindfulness practices, such as meditation and yoga, can be very helpful in this regard. Getting adequate sleep not only supports successful stress management, but also allows to body to get the rest it needs to function well. Reading personal development books can help define knowledge and skills on how to manage situations that may be new or uncomfortable to us. Seeking the support of a mental health professional can be very helpful in identifying healthy ways to manage stress specific to your situation.

MEDICATIONS

If you are particularly worried about your susceptibility to cancer, there are

---

20 Myrthala Moreno-Smith, Susan K Lutgendorf, and Anil K Sood, Impact of stress on cancer metastasis. Future Oncol. 2010 Dec; 6(12): 1863–1881.

a variety of cancer-suppressing medications that you can use. While some of them can be particularly potent cancer deterrents, they can be dangerous if used improperly. As with any drug, consult your physician before taking any of these medications, and be sure that you know about all of the side effects and potential risks.

For those with family histories of colon cancer, the Food and Drug Administration (FDA) recommends Celecoxib, most often known under the brand name 'Celebrex.' It works by disrupting the formation of polyps in your digestive tract, thus preventing cancer cells from growing there. However, those with histories of heart problems should be wary of using Celebrex. It is classified as a Non-Steroidal Anti-Inflammatory Drug (NSAID), and some NSAIDs can heighten your risk of heart disease and stroke.[21] In some patients, it may also cause serious gastrointestinal problems, including stomach ulcers.[22] Some studies suggest that aspirin may be an alternative for colon cancer risk reduction.

For breast cancer, there is a class of drugs known as selective estrogen response modifiers, or SERMs for short. In general, they have two primary functions; firstly, they are designed to suppress the production of estrogen in certain body tissues, particularly those in the breast. Secondly, they take on the functions that estrogen would normally fulfill, thus enabling your body to function properly without facilitating breast cancer growth.

But, like NSAIDs, SERMs have their own set of risks. Tamoxifen, for instance, heightens your risk of developing blood clots and having a stroke (though this risk is still relatively small). Tamoxifen can also exacerbate the symptoms of menopause, including hot flashes and vaginal dryness.[23]

---

21 The Internet Drug Index, "Celebrex." RxList, 2011. Web. http://www.rxlist.com/celebrex-drug.htm

22 Omudhome Ogbru, "Celebrex Side Effects Center." RxList, 2016. Web. http://www.rxlist.com/celebrex-side-effects-drug-center.htm

23 National Cancer Institute, "Hormone Therapy for Breast Cancer." 2012. Web. http://www.cancer.gov/cancertopics/factsheet/Therapy/hormone-therapy-breast

Tamoxifen has been shown to slightly increase the risk of uterine cancer, but for women who have a high risk for developing breast cancer, this risk is outweighed by its breast cancer reduction effects.

For postmenopausal women, an aromatase inhibitor called exemestane (brand name: Aromasin) is another alternative for medical breast cancer risk reduction. This drug may also be associated with menopausal symptoms, and also is associated with bone loss and thus may not be a good option for women with osteoporosis or osteopenia.

Prostate cancer patients have their own class of hormonal suppressant preventive agents, called 5α-reductase inhibitors. Two medications fall into this class of drugs, finasteride (brand name: Proscar) and dutasteride (Avodart). Similar to SERMs, they work by suppressing the production of androgens in the patient's body, thus preventing a cancer from growing. But, just like SERMS, these drugs may come with side effects.

Despite their side effects, these medications can be very useful for individuals with a high risk for a specific cancer, which underscores the importance of talking with your doctor about cancer risk assessment. If you are found to be at high risk, a cancer prevention specialist may offer you consultation to see if the benefits of a particular drug far outweigh its side effects in your particular case.

SURGICAL INTERVENTION

Preventive surgery is a last resort, as it can be stressful, risky and exceedingly expensive. It should only be used if your risk of developing cancer is high enough to justify it.

The most common form of preventive surgery is a bilateral mastectomy, the removal of one or both of your breasts. A mastectomy is often used to remove cancerous tissue in the breast, but it can also be used proactively to prevent the growth of cancer in that area. While a mastectomy will reduce the risk of breast cancer by a huge margin, it will not eliminate the risk altogether. Also, as you would expect, there are a variety of unrelated risks that come with the mastectomy procedure. Like any surgery, a mastectomy can lead to scarring, disfigurement, infection in the surgical area and blood clots. As such, only patients with an exceedingly high susceptibility to breast cancer should consider this option.

Similarly, prophylactic bilateral salpingo-oophorectomy (removal of both fallopian tubes and ovaries to prevent ovarian cancer) or prophylactic colectomy (removal of all or part of the colon to prevent colon cancer) may be considered in special high-risk patients.

These are just a few of the methods you can use to snuff out cancer before it grows. In short, the best way to minimize your chance of developing cancer is to take care of yourself. Have a keen awareness of what your body needs on a day-to-day basis, and act accordingly. Watch what you eat, keep track of your physical activity, and consult an experienced physician. If you'd like to learn more about the various types of cancer and what you can do to lower your own risk, please visit www.caprevinc.org or call 844-PREV-INC.

In summary, reducing your risk of getting cancer is possible. Start by understanding your family medical history as well as lifestyle and environmental risk factors. Have a positive attitude, a strict sense of self-awareness, and the willingness to change what you can and accept what you can't but with a proactive plan to manage your risk.

If you would like to know more about Dr. Melanie R. Palomares, M.D., M.S., and Cancer Prevention, Inc. please visit http://www.caprevinc.org/.

Branding
Small Business

RAYMOND AARON

B randing is an incredibly important tool for creating and building your
business. Large companies have been benefiting from branding ever since
people first started selling things to other people. Branding made those
businesses big.

If you're a small business owner, you probably imagine that small companies
are different and don't need branding as much as large companies do. Not
true. The truth is small businesses need branding just as much, if not more,
than large companies.

Perhaps you've thought about branding, but assumed you'd need millions of dollars to do it properly, or that branding is just the same thing as marketing. Nothing could be further from the truth.

Marketing is the engine of your company's success. Branding is the fuel in that engine.

In the old days, salespeople were a big part of the selling process. They recommended one product over another and laid out the reasons why it was better. Salespeople had credibility because they knew about all the products, and customers often took the advice they had to offer.

Today, consumers control the buying process. They shop in big box stores, super-sized supermarkets, and over the Internet — where there are no salespeople. Buyers now get online and gather information beforehand. They learn about all the products available and look to see if there really is any difference between them. Consumers also read reviews and check social media to see if both the company and the product are reputable. In other words, they want to know what the brand is all about.

The way of commerce used to be: "Nothing happens till something is sold." Today it's: "Nothing happens till something is branded!"

DEFINING A BRAND

A brand is a proper name that stands for something. It lives in the consumer's mind, has positive or negative characteristics, and invokes a feeling or an image. In short, it's a person's perception of a product or a company.

When all goes well, consumers associate the same characteristics with a brand that the company talks about in its advertising, public relations, marketing and sales materials. Of course, when a product doesn't live up to what the company says about it, the brand gets a bad reputation. On the other hand, if a product or service over-delivers on the promises made, the brand can become a superstar.

RECOGNIZING BRANDING AND ITS CHARACTERISTICS

Branding is the science and art of making something that isn't unique, unique. Branding in the marketplace is the same as branding on a ranch. On a ranch, ranchers use branding to differentiate their cattle from every other rancher's cattle (because all cattle look pretty much the same). In the marketplace, branding is what makes a product stand out in a crowd of similar products. The right branding gets you noticed, remembered and sold — or perhaps I should say bought, because today it is all about buying, not selling.

There are four main characteristics of branding that make it an integral part of the marketing and purchasing process.

1. Branding makes you trustworthy and known

Branding makes a product more special than other products. With branding, a normal, everyday product has a personality, and a first and last name, and people know who you are.

In today's marketplace, most products are, more or less, just like their competition. Toilet paper is toilet paper, milk is milk, and a grocery store by any other name is still a grocery store. However, branding takes a product and makes it unique. For example, high-quality drinking water is available from just about every tap in the Western world and it's free, but people pay good money for it when it comes in a bottle. Branding takes bottled water and makes Evian.

Furthermore, every aspect of your brand gives potential customers a feeling or comfort level that they associate with you. The more powerful and positive that feeling is, the more easily and more frequently they will want to do business with you and, indeed, will do business with you.

2. Branding differentiates you from others

Strong branding makes you better than your competition, and makes your product name memorable and easy to remember. Even if your product is absolutely the same as every other product like it, branding makes it special. Branding makes it the first product a consumer thinks about when deciding to make a purchase.

Branding also makes a product seem popular. Everyone knows about it, which implicitly says people like it. And, if people like it, it must be good.

3. Branding makes you worth more money

The stronger your branding is, the more likely people are willing to spend that little bit extra because they believe you, your product, your service, or your business are worth it. They may say they won't, but they will. They do it all the time.

For example, a one-pound box of Godiva chocolates costs about $40; the same weight of Hershey's Kisses costs about $4. The quality of the chocolate isn't ten times greater. The reason people buy Godiva is that the brand Godiva means "gift" whereas the brand Hershey means "snack". Gifts obviously cost more than snacks.

4. Branding pre-sells your product

In the buying age, people most often make the decision on which products to pick up before they walk into the store. The stronger the branding, the more likely people are to think in terms of your product rather than the product category. For example, people are as likely, maybe even more likely, to add Hellmann's to the shopping list as they are to write down simply mayo. The same is true for soda, ketchup, and many other products with successful, strong branding.

Plus, as soon as a shopper gets to the shelf, branding can provide a quick reminder of what products to grab in a few ways:

- An icon or logo
- A specific color
- An audio icon

BRANDING IN A SMALL BUSINESS

Big companies spend millions of dollars on advertising, marketing, and public relations (PR) to build recognition of a new product name. They get their selling messages out to the public using television, radio, magazines, and the Internet. They can even throw money at damage control when necessary. The strategies for branding are the same in a small business, but the scale, costs, and a few of the tactics change.

Make your brand name work harder

The name of a small business can mean everything in terms of branding. Your brand name needs to work harder for your business than you do. It's the first thing a prospective customer sees, and it is how they will remember you. A brand name has to be memorable when spoken, and focused in its meaning. If the name doesn't represent what consumers believe about a product and the company that makes it, then that brand will fail.

In building your product's reputation and image, less is often significantly more. Make sure the name you choose immediately gives a sense of what you do.

Large corporations have millions of dollars to take a meaningless brand name and make it stand for something. Small businesses don't, so use words that really mean something. Strive for something interesting and be right on point. You don't need to be boring.

Plumbers, for example, would do well setting themselves apart with names like "The On-Time Plumber" or "24/7 Plumbing". The same is true for electricians, IT providers, or even marketing consultants. Plenty of other types of business are so general in nature they just don't work hard enough in a business or product name.

Even the playing field: The Net

The Internet has leveled the playing field for small businesses like nothing else. You can use the Internet in several ways to market your brand:

Website: Developing and maintaining a website is easier than ever. Anyone can find your business regardless of its size.

Social Media: Facebook and Twitter can promote your brand in a cost-effective manner.

BUILDING YOUR BRAND WITH THE BRANDING LADDER

Even if you do everything perfectly the first time (and I don't know anyone who does), branding takes time. How much time isn't just up to you, but you can speed things along by understanding the different levels of branding, as well as the business and marketing strategies that can get you to the top.

Introducing the Branding Ladder

Moving through the levels of branding is like climbing a ladder to the top of the marketplace. The Branding Ladder has five distinct rungs and, unlike stairs, you can't take them two at a time. You have to take them in order, and some businesses spend more time on each rung than others.

You can also think of the Branding Ladder in terms of a scale from zero to ten. Everyone starts at zero. If you properly climb the ladder, you can end up at 12 out of 10. The Branding Ladder below shows a special rung at the top of the ladder that can take your business over the top. The following section explains the Branding Ladder and how your small business can move up it.

THE BRANDING LADDER	
Brand Advocacy	12/10
Brand Insistence	10/10
Brand Preference	3/10
Brand Awareness	1/10
Brand Absence	0/10

Rung 1: Living in the void

Your business, in fact every business, starts at the bottom rung, which is called brand absence, meaning you have no brand whatsoever except your own name. On a scale of one to ten, brand absence is, of course, zero. That's the worst place to live and obviously the most difficult entrepreneurially. The good news is that the only way is up.

Ninety-seven percent of businesses live on this rung of the Branding Ladder. They earn far less than they want to earn, far less than they should earn, and far less than they would earn if they did exactly the same work under a real brand.

Rung 2: Achieving awareness

Brand awareness is a good first step up the ladder to the second rung. Actually, it's really good, especially because 97 percent of businesses never get there. You want people to be aware of you. When person A speaks to person B and says, "Have you heard of "The 24/7 Plumber?" You want the answer to be "yes".

On that scale of one to ten, however, brand awareness is only a one. It's better than nothing, but not that much better. Although people know of your brand, being aware doesn't mean that they are interested in buying it. Coca Cola drinkers know about Pepsi, but they don't drink it.

Rung 3: Becoming the preferred brand

Getting to the third rung, brand preference, is definitely a real step up. This rung means that people prefer to use your product or service rather than that of your competition. They believe there is a real difference between you and others, and you're their first choice. This rung is a crucial branding stage for parity products, such as bottled water and breakfast cereals, not to mention plumbers, electricians, lawyers, and all the others. Brand preference is clearly better than brand awareness, but it's less than halfway up the ladder.

Car rental companies represent a perfect example of why brand preference may not be enough. When someone lands at an airport and needs to rent a car on the spot, he or she may go straight to the preferred rental counter. If that company has a car available, it's a sale. However, if all the cars for that company have been rented, the person will move to the next rental kiosk without much thought, because one rental car is just as good as another.

Exerting Brand Preference needs to be easy and convenient

If all you have is brand preference, your business is on shaky ground and you can lose business for the feeblest of reasons. Very few people go to a second or third supermarket just to find their favorite brand of bottled water. Similarly, a shopper may prefer one store over another but, if both stores sell the same products, he or she will often go to the closest store even if it is not the better liked one. The reason for staying nearby does not need to be a dramatic one — the shopper may simply be tired, on a tight schedule, or not in the mood to travel.

Rung 4: Making it you and only you

When your customers are so committed to your product or service that they won't accept a substitute, you have reached the fourth rung of the Branding Ladder. All companies strive to reach this place, called brand insistence.

Brand insistence means that someone's experience with a product in terms of performance, durability, customer service, and image has been sufficiently exceptional. As a result, the product has earned an incredible level of loyalty.

If the product isn't available where the customer is, he or she will literally not buy something else. Rather, the person will look for the preferred product elsewhere. Can you imagine what a fabulous place this is for a company to be? Brand insistence is the best of the best, the perfect ten out of ten, the whole ball of wax.

Apple is a perfect example of brand insistence

Apple users don't just think, they know in their heads and hearts, that anything made by Apple is technologically-advanced, user-friendly, and just all-around superior. Committed to everything Apple, Mac users won't even entertain the thought that a PC may have positive attributes.

Apple people love everything about their Macs, iPads, iPhones, the Mac stores and all those apps. When the company introduces a new product, many of its brand-insistent fans actually wait in line overnight to be one of the first to have it. Steve Jobs is one of their idols.

Considering one big potential problem

Unfortunately, you can lose brand insistence much more quickly than you can achieve it. Brand-insistent customers have such high expectations that they can be disillusioned or disappointed by just one bad product experience. You also have to consistently reinforce the positives because insistence can fade over time. Even someone who has bought and re-bought a specific brand of car for the last 20 years can decide it's just time for a change. That's how fickle the world is.

At ten out of ten, brand insistence may seem like the top rung of the ladder, but it's not. One rung is actually better, and it involves getting your brand-insistent customers to keep polishing your brand for you.

Rung 5: Getting customers to do the work for you

Brand advocacy is the highest rung on the ladder. It's better than ten out of ten because you have customers who are so happy with your product that they want everyone to know about it and use it. Think of them as uber-fans. Not only do they recommend you to friends and family, they also practically shout your praises from the rooftops, interrupt conversations among strangers to give their opinion, and tell everyone they meet how fantastic you are. Most companies can only aspire to this level of customer satisfaction. Apple is one of the few large corporations in recent history that has brand advocates all over the world.

- Brand advocacy does the following five extraordinary things for your company. Brand advocacy:

- Provides a level of visibility that you couldn't pay for if you tried. Brand advocates are so enthusiastic they talk about you all the time, and reach people in ways general media and public relations can't. You get great visibility because they make sure people actually listen.

- Delivers free advertising and public relations. Companies love the extra super-positive messaging, all for free.

- Affords a level of credibility that literally can't be bought. Brand advocates are more than just walking testimonials. They are living proof that you are the best.

- Provides pre-sold prospective customers. Advocate recommendations carry so much weight that they are worth much more than plain referrals. They deliver customers ready and committed to purchasing your product or service.

- Increases profits exponentially. Brand advocates are money-making machines for your business because they increase sales and decrease marketing costs.

For these reasons, brand advocacy is 12 out of 10!!

BRANDING YOURSELF: HOW TO DO SO IN FOUR EASY WAYS

If you're interested in branding your product or company, you may not be sure where to begin. The good news: I'm here to help. You can brand in many ways, but here I pare it down to four ways to help you start:

Branding by association

This way involves hanging out with and being seen with people who are very much higher than you in your particular niche.

Branding by achievement

This way repurposes your previous achievements.

Branding by testimonial

This way makes use of the testimonials that you receive but have likely never used.

Branding by WOW

A WOW is the pleasantly unexpected, the equivalent of going the extra mile. The easiest and most certain way to WOW people is to tell them that you've written a book. To discover how you can write a book of own, go to www.BrandingSmallBusinessForDummies.com.

Happiness: How to Experience the "Real Deals"

MARCI SHIMOFF

I was 41 years old, stretched out on a lounge chair by my pool and reflecting on my life. I had achieved all that I thought I needed to be happy.

You see, when I was a child, I thought there would be five main things that would ensure that I'd be happy: a successful career helping people, a loving husband, a comfortable home, a great body, and a wonderful circle of friends. After years of study, hard work, and a few "lucky breaks," I finally had them all. (Okay, so my body didn't quite look like Halle Berry's—but four out of five isn't bad!) You think I'd have been on the top of the world.

But surprisingly I wasn't. I felt an emptiness inside that the outer successes of life couldn't fill. I was also afraid that if I lost any of those things, I might be miserable. Sadly, I knew I wasn't alone in feeling this way.

While happiness is the one thing we all truly want, so few people really experience the deep and lasting fulfillment that fills our soul. Why aren't we finding it?

Because, in the words of the old country western song, we're looking for happiness in "all the wrong places."

Looking around, I saw that the happiest people I knew weren't the most successful and famous. Some were married, some were single. Some had lots of money, and some didn't have a dime. Some of them even had health challenges. From where I stood, there seemed to be no rhyme or reason to what made people happy. The obvious question became: *Could a person actually be happy for no reason?*

I had to find out.

So I threw myself into the study of happiness. I interviewed scores of scientists, as well as 100 unconditionally happy people. (I call them the Happy 100.) I delved into the research from the burgeoning field of positive psychology, the study of the positive traits that enable people to enjoy meaningful, fulfilling, and happy lives.

What I found changed my life. To share this knowledge with others, I wrote a book called *Happy for No Reason: 7 Steps to Being Happy from the Inside Out.*

One day, as I sat down to compile my findings, all the pieces of the puzzle fell into place. I had a simple, but profound "a-ha"—there's a continuum of happiness:

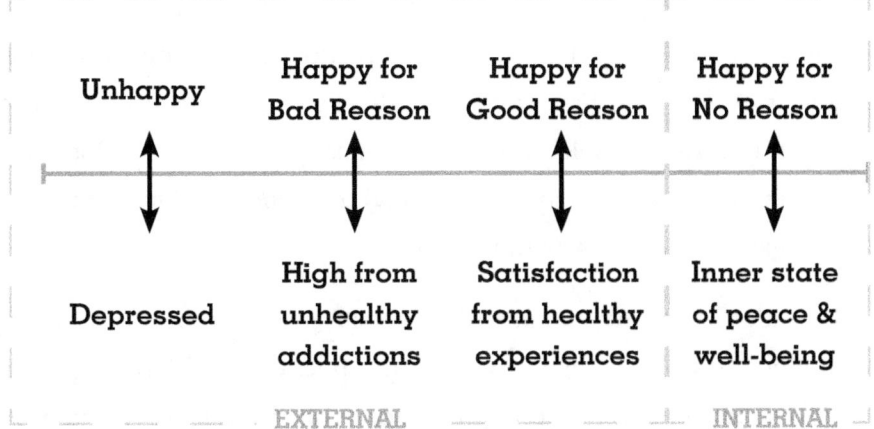

Unhappy: We all know what this means: life seems flat. Some of the signs are anxiety, fatigue, feeling blue or low—your "garden-variety" unhappiness. This isn't the same as clinical depression, which is characterized by deep despair and hopelessness that dramatically interferes with your ability to live a normal life, and for which professional help is absolutely necessary.

Happy for Bad Reason: When people are unhappy, they often try to make themselves feel better by indulging in addictions or behaviors that may feel good in the moment but are ultimately detrimental. They seek the highs that come from drugs, alcohol, excessive sex, "retail therapy," compulsive gambling, over-eating, and too much television-watching, to name a few. This kind of "happiness" is hardly happiness at all. It is only a temporary way to numb or escape our unhappiness through fleeting experiences of pleasure.

Happy for Good Reason: This is what people usually mean by happiness: having good relationships with our family and friends, success in our careers, financial security, a nice house or car, or using our talents and strengths well. It's the pleasure we derive from having the healthy things in our lives that we want.

Don't get me wrong. I'm all for this kind of happiness! It's just that it's only half the story. Being Happy for Good Reason depends on the external conditions of our lives—these conditions change or are lost, our happiness usually goes too. Relying solely on this type of happiness is where a lot of our fear is stemming from these days. We're afraid the things we think we need to be happy may be slipping from our grasp.

Deep inside, I think we all know that life isn't meant to be about getting by, numbing our pain, or having everything "under control." True happiness doesn't come from merely collecting an assortment of happy experiences. At our core, we know there's something more than this.

There is. It's the next level on the happiness continuum—Happy for No Reason.

Happy for No Reason: This is true happiness—a state of peace and well-being that isn't dependent on external circumstances.

Happy for No Reason isn't elation, euphoria, mood spikes, or peak experiences that don't last. It doesn't mean grinning like a fool 24/7 or experiencing a superficial high. Happy for No Reason isn't an emotion. In fact, when you are Happy for No Reason, you can have *any* emotion—including sadness, fear, anger or hurt—but you still experience that underlying state of peace and well-being.

When you're Happy for No Reason, you *bring* happiness to your outer experiences rather than trying to *extract* happiness from them. You don't need to manipulate the world around you to try to make yourself happy. You live from happiness, rather than *for* happiness.

This is a revolutionary concept. Most of us focus on being Happy for Good Reason, stringing together as many happy experiences as we can, like beads in a necklace, to create a happy life. We have to spend a lot of time and energy trying to find just the right beads so we can have a "happy necklace".

Being Happy for No Reason, in our necklace analogy, is like having a happy string. No matter what beads we put on our necklace—good, bad or indifferent—our inner experience, which is the string that runs through them all, is happy, and creates a happy life.

Happy for No Reason is a state that's been spoken of in virtually all spiritual and religious traditions throughout history. The concept is universal. In Buddhism, it is called causeless joy; in Christianity, the kingdom of Heaven within; and in Judaism it is called *ashrei*, an inner sense of holiness and health. In Islam it is called *falah*, happiness and well-being; and in Hinduism it is called *ananda*, or pure bliss. Some traditions refer to it as an enlightened or awakened state.

So how can you be Happy for No Reason?

Science is verifying the way. Researchers in the field of positive psychology have found that we each have a "happiness set-point," that determines our level of happiness. No matter what happens, whether it's something as exhilarating as winning the lottery or as challenging as a horrible accident, most people eventually return to their original happiness level. Like your weight set-point, which keeps the scale hovering around the same number, your happiness set-point will remain the same **unless you make a concerted effort to change it.** In the same way you'd crank up the thermostat to get comfortable on a chilly day, you actually have the power to reprogram your happiness set-point to a higher level of peace and well-being. The secret lies in practicing the habits of happiness.

Some books and programs will tell you that you can simply decide to be happy. They say just make up your mind to be happy—and you will be.

I don't agree.

You can't just decide to be happy, any more than you can decide to be fit or to be a great piano virtuoso and expect instant mastery. You can, however, decide to take the necessary steps, like exercising or taking piano lessons—and by practicing those skills, you can get in shape or give recitals. In the same way, you can become Happy for No Reason through practicing the habits of happy people.

All of your habitual thoughts and behaviors in the past have created specific neural pathways in the wiring in your brain, like grooves in a record. When we think or behave a certain way over and over, the neural pathway is strengthened and the groove becomes deeper—the way a well-traveled route through a field eventually becomes a clear-cut path. Unhappy people tend to have more negative neural pathways. This is why you can't just ignore the realities of your brain's wiring and *decide* to be happy! To raise your level of happiness, you have to create new grooves.

Scientists used to think that once a person reached adulthood, the brain was fairly well "set in stone" and there wasn't much you could do to change it. But new research is revealing exciting information about the brain's neuroplasticity: when you think, feel and act in different ways, the brain changes and actually rewires itself. You aren't doomed to the same negative neural pathways for your whole life. Leading brain researcher Dr. Richard Davidson, of the University of Wisconsin says, "Based on what we know of the plasticity of the brain, we can think of things like happiness and compassion as skills that are no different from learning to play a musical instrument or tennis .... it is possible to train our brains to be happy."

While a few of the Happy 100 I interviewed were born happy, most of them learned to be happy by practicing habits that supported their happiness. That means wherever you are on the happiness continuum, it's entirely in your power to raise your happiness level.

In the course of my research, I uncovered 21 core happiness habits that anyone can use to become happier and stay that way. You can find all 21 happiness habits at www.HappyForNoReason.com

Here are a few tips to get you started:

1. **Incline Your Mind Toward Joy.** Have you noticed that your mind tends to register the negative events in your life more than the positive? If you get ten compliments in a day and one criticism, what do you remember? For most people, it's the criticism. Scientists call this our "negativity bias" — our primitive survival wiring that causes us to pay more attention to the negative than the positive. To reverse this bias, get into the daily habit of consciously registering the positive around you: the sun on your skin, the taste of a favorite food, a smile or kind word from a co-worker or friend. Once you notice something positive, take a moment to savor it deeply and feel it; make it more than just a mental observation. Spend 20 seconds soaking up the happiness you feel.

2. **Let Love Lead.** One way to power up your heart's flow is by sending loving kindness to your friends and family, as well as strangers you pass on the street. Next time you're waiting for the elevator at work, stuck in a line at the store or caught up in traffic, send a silent wish to the people you see for their happiness, well-being, and health. Simply wishing others well switches on the "pump" in your own heart that generates love and creates a strong current of happiness.

3. **Lighten Your Load.** To make a habit of letting go of worries and negative thoughts, start by letting go on the physical level. Cultural anthropologist Angeles Arrien recommends giving or throwing away 27 items a day for nine days. This deceptively simple practice will help you break attachments that no longer serve you.

4. **Make Your Cells Happy.** Your brain contains a veritable pharmacopeia of natural happiness-enhancing neurochemicals — endorphins, serotonin, oxytocin, and dopamine — just waiting to be released to every organ and cell in your body. The way that you eat, move, rest, and even your facial expression can shift the balance of your body's feel-good-chemicals, or "Joy Juice", in your favor. To dispense some extra Joy Juice — smile. Scientists have discovered that smiling decreases stress hormones and boosts happiness chemicals, which increase the body's T-cells, reduce pain, and enhance relaxation. You may not feel like it, but smiling — even artificially to begin with — starts the ball rolling and will turn into a real smile in short order.

5. **Hang with the Happy.** We catch the emotions of those around us just like we catch their colds — it's called emotional contagion. So it's important to make wise choices about the company you keep. Create appropriate boundaries with emotional bullies and "happiness vampires" who suck the life out of you. Develop your happiness "dream team" — a mastermind or support group you meet with regularly to keep you steady on the path of raising your happiness.

"Happily ever after" isn't just for fairytales or for only the lucky few. Imagine experiencing inner peace and well-being as the backdrop for everything else in your life. When you're Happy for No Reason, it's not that your life always looks perfect — it's that, however it looks, you'll still be happy!

By Marci Shimoff. Based on the New York Times bestseller *Happy for No Reason: 7 Steps to Being Happy from the Inside Out*, which offers a revolutionary approach to experiencing deep and lasting happiness. The woman's face of the *Chicken Soup for the Soul* series and a featured teacher in *The Secret*, Marci is an authority on success, happiness, and the law of attraction. To order *Happy for No Reason* and receive free bonus gifts, go to www.happyfornoreason.com/mybook.

Sex, Love and Relationships

DR. JOHN GRAY

Just as great sex is important to lasting love, good health is important to sex and relationships. About 12 years ago, I cured myself of early stage Parkinson's disease. The doctors were amazed, but my wife was even more amazed. She noted that our relationship and sex life had become dramatically better. It turns out that the natural supplements I used to reverse Parkinson's can also make you more attentive and loving in your relationship. At that point, I realized that good relationship skills alone were not enough to sustain love and passion for a lifetime.

I shared many insights gained from my 40 years' experience as a marriage counselor and coach in *Men Are From Mars, Women Are From Venus*. And while my insights go a long way towards helping men and women understand and support each other, good communication skills alone are not always enough. For better relationships, we not only need to be healthy, but we must also experience optimum brain function.

If you are tired, depressed, anxious, not sleeping well, or in pain, then certainly romantic feelings will become a thing of the past. My recovery from Parkinson's revealed to me the profound connection between the quality of our health and our relationships. This insight has motivated me, over the past twelve years, to research the secrets of optimum health as a foundation for lasting love.

These are health secrets that are generally not explored in medical school. In medical school, doctors are indoctrinated into the culture of examining the symptoms, identifying the sickness, and prescribing a drug to treat that sickness. They learn very little about how to be healthy or to sustain successful relationships.

There are no university courses entitled "Better Nutrition For Better Sex". Drugs sometimes save lives, but they also have negative side effects that do little to preserve the passion in a relationship. Ideally, drugs should be used as a last resort and 90 % of our health plan should be drug free. From this perspective, the heath care crisis, as well as our high rate of divorce in America, is indirectly caused by our dependence on doctors and prescription drugs.

Most people have not even considered that taking prescribed drugs (even for the small stuff) can weaken their relationships, which in turn makes them more vulnerable to more disease. For example, if you are feeling depressed or anxious, a drug may numb your pain, but it does nothing to help you correct the cause of your problem. It can even prevent you from feeling your natural motivation to get the emotional support you need. In a variety of ways, our common health complaints are all expressions of two major conditions: our lack of education to identify and support unmet gender-specific emotional needs; and our lack of education to identify and support unmet gender-specific nutritional needs.

With an understanding of natural solutions that have been around for thousands of years, drugs are not needed to treat many common complaints. Some symptoms like low energy, weight gain, allergies, hormonal imbalance, mood swings, poor sleep, indigestion, lack of focus, ADD and ADHD, procrastination, low motivation, memory loss, decreased libido, PMS, vaginal dryness, muscle and joint pain, or the lack of passion in life and/or our relationships can be treated drug-free. By using drugs (even over-the-counter drugs) to treat these common complaints, our bodies and relationships are weakened, making us more vulnerable to bigger and more costly health challenges like cancer, diabetes, heart disease, auto-immune disease, dementia, and Alzheimer's. In simple terms, by handling the easy stuff (the common complaints) without doctors and drugs, we can protect ourselves from the big stuff (cancer, heart disease, dementia, etc.) We can be healthy and also enjoy lasting love and passion in our personal lives.

Even if you are taking anti-depressants or hormone replacement therapy, sometimes all it takes to stop treating the symptom is to directly handle the cause. With specific mineral orotates (something most people have never heard of) or omega three oil from the brains of salmon, your stress levels immediately drop and you begin to feel happy and in love again.

For every health challenge, we have explored the effects on our relationships, with as well as natural remedies that can sometimes produce immediate positive results. You can find these natural solutions to common health complaints for free at my website: www.MarsVenus.com.

What they don't teach in medical school is how to be healthy and happy without the use of drugs or hormone replacement. By refusing drugs and taking responsibility for your health, a wealth of new possibilities can become available to you. We are designed to be healthy and happy, and it is within our reach if we commit to increasing our knowledge.

New research regarding the brain differences in men and women reveals how specific nutritional supplements, combined with gender-specific relationship and self-nurturing skills, can stimulate the hormones of health, happiness and increased energy. Over the past 10 years in my healing center in California, I witnessed how natural solutions coupled with gender-specific relationship skills could solve our common health complaints without drugs. By addressing these common complaints without prescribed drugs, not only do we feel better, but our relationships have the potential to improve dramatically.

Ultimately the cause of all our common complaints is higher stress levels. Researchers around the world all agree that chronic stress levels in our bodies provide a basis for any and all disease to take hold. An easy and quick solution for lowering our stress reactions is specific nutritional support combined with gender-smart relationship skills. Extra nutritional support is needed because stress depletes the body very quickly of essential nutrients. When a car engine is running more quickly, it uses fuel more quickly. When we are stressed, we need both extra nutrients and extra emotional support. Understanding what we need to take and where to get it requires education. Every week day at www.MarsVenus.com I have a live daily show where I freely answer questions and provide this much-needed new gender-specific insight.

At www.MarsVenus.com, we are happy to share what we have learned for creating healthy bodies and positive relationships. You can find a host of natural solutions for common complaints and feel confident that you have the power to feel fully alive with an abundance of energy and positive feelings that will enrich all your relationships.

The Modern Healer

Herman Siu
& Martin Siu

G ood health is a God-given right; it's our birthright. Yet, while we have made huge technological advances to facilitate cross-planet communication in real-time, we haven't been as progressive in keeping ourselves healthy.

We may be living longer but, tragically, children are dying from cancers, diabetes is on the rise, and young adults are suddenly getting heart attacks. Chronic fatigue, depression, and anxiety assail us. We rely on drugs to fix our health problems and we spend billions of dollars on prescriptions that may alleviate the symptoms but leave the root cause untouched. In our fast-paced societies, we have lost the connection with nature and the natural elements that make up our bodies. Surely, there is an alternative way to heal ourselves, or even to prevent disease from occurring in the first place.

The long and short of it is that we don't have to drop out of society and reside in the woods to live happier and healthier lives. The answer to good health and longevity lies right at our fingertips – in the air we breathe, the foods we eat, and water we drink. That's the best prescription for the Modern Healer, and these are the guiding principles we use in our healing practice. As 5th and 6th generation healers immersed in traditions that date back to ancient Chinese Shaolin practices, we adhere to the disciplined and holistic approach of our forefathers.

We believe that a body in full balance has everything it needs to fight off disease, stay and look young, and be active and involved, regardless of the biological age. This belief has been supported by patient outcomes through successive centuries of practice by the healers in our family. We share this knowledge with you to empower you as a Modern Healer, so that you may take control of and assume responsibility for your own health and be the expert in your own healing and wellness journey.

To be empowered as a Modern Healer, you must first understand the core concepts of energy or Qi (chi) as defined by ancient Chinese healing texts.

Dr. Paul Unschuld, a highly-regarded authority on Chinese medicine and multi-book author said, "The core Chinese concept of qi bears no resemblance to the Western concept of 'energy'. We perceive that there is a knowledge gap in the current understanding of eastern medicine in the western world. Mindful of the wisdom suggested by the Chinese proverb, "A journey of a thousand miles begins with a single step," we have written this chapter as our first step towards bridging that divide.

There are three primary components to balance Qi. Qi is a fundamental power underlying all of nature, and it is a vital life force that runs through our body. There are three primary components to balance our Qi. The first component to boosting our Qi is the air we breathe, the second is the food we eat, and the third is the water we drink.

AIR GIVES LIFE

Almost all of life needs oxygen to survive. We take in oxygen from our surroundings to harness energy and use it to power the inner workings of our bodies.

In the Huangdi Neijing, the ancient Chinese foundation medical text, the lungs breathe in what's known as, da qi, or "great qi.". Once we breathe in the air, the lungs extract the Qi from the da qi. Based on this understanding, we perceive that Qi relates to life-sustaining oxygen.

What is the secret to having great Qi? It is the harmonization of the mind, body, and spirit.

In martial arts, we use our mind to harness Qi by controlling our breath. We use our body to breathe, and we put our bodies through constant practice to master our Qi. Once it has been mastered, the Qi can be at our fingertips in a moment's notice. We call it in this form the spirit.

Viewed from this perspective, it's simple to make the most of living and get the best use of your life. The first step to taking back control of your health is by learning to breathe correctly.

Notice, right this moment, how you are breathing. Are you breathing from your diaphragm or the stomach, or are you taking in quick snatches of air? The majority of us take shallow breaths because we have forgotten how to breathe deeply and fully, and the only time we do so is when we are in yoga or meditation. Having become a society of superficial breathers, we are not benefitting from the fact that 70% of the toxins in our bodies are released through breath. By breathing shallowly, we are shortchanging ourselves because hypoxia, or insufficient oxygen in the body's cells, has been linked to degenerative diseases.

Remember, breath equals life and a long breath enhances a long life. Breathing correctly is your first responsibility as a Modern Healer.

FOOD FOR HEALING

The second primary component to balance our Qi is food.

The ancient Greek physician, Hippocrates, who is widely known as the "Father of Medicine", is quoted as saying "Let food be thy medicine and medicine be thy food." Fast forward several centuries; Dr. Roger J. Williams, who discovered the B-vitamin, said in 1971, "The human body heals itself and nutrition provides the resources to accomplish the task." The Chinese are well known to eat their food in its season. For example, no watermelon is eaten in winter since it grows in the hot summer climate.

It is empowering to discover that we need look no further than our own gardens and our kitchens to find healing nutrition that supports health for our family. By making healthy food choices, we ensure that we age gracefully and live out the rest of the twilight years harmoniously and peacefully, without the blight of Alzheimer's, dementia, or other failing diseases.

"So many people spend their health gaining wealth & then have to spend their wealth to regain their health." - Chinese proverb

Our philosophy is that, with right air, right food and right water (in this order), you detoxify naturally, without having to go on rigid short-term fasts.

With the right balance of foods that are appropriate to your body type, you'll get rid of excess fat and flab, find the correct body weight, be brimming over with energy, have the mental clarity to solve challenges with ease, and be in love with your life.

If you're tired of feeling frustrated, angry, depressed, unsure, overweight, tired, and in despair, look to your shopping list, refrigerator and kitchen closets for the culprits. Are they full of processed foods and refined sugars? Are you eating natural grains, green leafy vegetables and fresh fruit?

In this chapter, we'll draw on healing secrets that we share with our clients in our Toronto-based clinic. We'll discuss the major foods that prevent inflammation, help you recover from cuts and wounds, and help detoxify the system.

But for the Modern Healer, the first line of defense is maintaining a healthy pH balance. Acid is corrosive and is the biggest culprit of many degenerative and deadly diseases. It's true that some acid is needed in the body. The stomach uses it to break down the food we eat into macronutrients such as proteins, fats and carbohydrates, and micronutrients such as vitamins and minerals that it may be easily absorbed by the body. But most typical diets are packed with sugar, animal proteins, and processed foods.

WHY PH BALANCE IS CRUCIAL TO GOOD HEALTH

The pH is a measure of acidity or alkalinity. The billions of cells that make up our bodies need an alkaline environment to function, to stay healthy, and to regenerate. Too much acid in our bodies creates ripe conditions for the growth of bacteria, yeast, fungus, viruses, mold and other diseases. Cells that are starved of oxygen are unable to regenerate. Once starved, they are unable to repair damage or rid the body of noxious chemicals and toxins. In time, the cells die; research now points out that cancer is the result of an over-acidic body. An ideal balance for our bodies is measured between a pH of 7.2 – 7.4. You can measure this by dipping pH testing strips into a sample of saliva or urine. An acidic body will produce a pH reading of less than 7.2, which means there is a lack of oxygenation at the cellular level. Your body may even create more fat cells to store the corrosive acid, leading to unwanted weight gain. If the body is malnourished or lacking any Alkaline minerals, it goes in search of calcium to optimize the pH level, and extracts calcium from your bones (joints), teeth and tissues which in turn leaves the bones weak. Calcium is one of the most important alkaline minerals as it increases the oxygen level in the blood. This calcium depletion results in arthritis and osteoporosis. In the initial stages of over-acidity, you may suffer from joint pains, headaches, and weight gain. In an acidic state, the body is trying to expel excess acid through your skin, causing muscle cramps, eczema, acne, swelling, irritation, and general aches and pains. People in this state get grouchier and irritable, and they age faster than those with a balanced pH body. Other so-called modern diseases linked to an acidic body include diabetes, osteoarthritis, acid reflux, irritable bowel syndrome, premature aging, muscle and chronic fatigue, bone loss and osteoporosis.

"The only way to keep good health is to eat what you don't want, drink what you don't like, & do what you'd rather not" -Chinese proverb

GETTING YOUR PH BALANCE RIGHT THROUGH FOODS

Our experience has shown that a balanced diet should be 85-90% alkaline and 10-15% acidic. Body functions and hand-eye coordination work at their optimal state at these levels. It's better for the body to be slightly alkaline than it is to be slightly acidic. Now that we understand why the pH balance is the first line of defense and why it's crucial to maintain the correct pH balance, let's explore quickly what foods contribute to a more alkaline state and more acidic state. A food is classified as alkaline or acidic according to its mineral content. Alkaline-forming foods contain more minerals such as calcium, magnesium, manganese, iron, and potassium. Some acid-promoting minerals include phosphorous, copper, and sulfur. Carbonated drinks are acid forming because they are loaded with sugar and phosphorus, which can lead to weight gain. Have a healthy serving of kale or broccoli instead, which nourishes your body with helpful calcium and magnesium for bone and muscle health. Alkaline foods include apples, apricots, cantaloupes, cauliflower, broccoli, kale, almonds, chestnuts and walnuts. The complete list is much longer and we will examine the healing qualities of alkaline-based nutrition in the section under Anti-Inflammation Foods. Acidic foods include ice-cream, manufactured processed foods with refined sugar, meat, fish, poultry, and eggs. This is not to say that all fruits and vegetables are alkaline. Some are in fact very acidic. Acidic vegetables include corn, onions, and garlic. In the fruit category will fall cranberries, blueberries, and currants. As you grow older, it's harder to expel the acid that is in your body. The longer acid exists, the more it will congeal and the more it will attack your cells and immune system. Acidic conditions manifest one illness at a time. Symptoms include arthritis, muscle fatigue, and body aches. At the point that you are weakest is when you're most prone to infections and diseases because infections live off acidic waste products. At our clinic, we will examine the root cause of your health problems, not just the symptoms. We will customize a holistic healing plan drawing on our experience and expertise to restore you to the right balance, homeostasis, so you may live your life in joy and harmony.

"Tell me and I'll forget; show me and I may remember; involve me and I'll understand" - Chinese proverb

ALKALINE AND ANTI-INFLAMMATION FOODS

Inflammation is a natural body response to injury. You bruise when you hit your shin against a table leg or when you sprain an ankle. Chronic inflammation, if undetected, can result in debilitating illnesses such as heart disease, cancer, diabetes, arthritis, and Alzheimer's. Fried and processed foods, as well as foods that contain trans-fat, increase the risk of inflammation. We've mentioned that alkaline foods prevent inflammation, and these are ordinary fruits, vegetables, and herbs that you can find in your refrigerator, spice cabinet, and even in your own garden. There are many creative ways to prepare these foods for a delicious, nutritious, beneficial anti-inflammation diet/alkaline diet. Here is a small list of foods to keep your body in balance and in good health.

Avocados: they contain healthy fats, phyto-proteins, vitamins, minerals and dietary fiber that is sorely lacking in the western societies. Low in sugar content, avocados may help to lower cholesterol levels, and increase resistance to diabetes, coronary heart disease, stroke and cancer, while promoting a healthy body weight and body mass index (BMI). Avocados are best eaten fresh.

Bamboo shoots: which is not a common vegetable on the western table, were identified by the Compendium of Materia Medica, the most comprehensive medical book in the history of traditional Chinese Medicine. Bamboo shoots promote the circulatory system, supplementing the body's natural energy, and are recommended as a daily dish. A traditional forest vegetable in Chinese diets for 2,500 years, nutrient-rich bamboo shoots are being shown in modern research to help prevent cancer, and to aid in weight loss, digestion, and the appetite.

Bamboo shoots are rich in essential amino acids and fatty acids and, because of their low sugar content, they are useful for treating hypertension, hyperlipemia, and hyperglycemia.

Broccoli: just about all vegetables are good, but some are more alkaline than others. Broccoli counts among the latter as it is rich in important vitamins such as A, C, K, B-complex and minerals including iron, zinc, and phosphorus. Broccoli is also rich in phytonutrients, which are natural chemicals that help protect plants and prevent disease in our bodies.

Broccoli helps to prevent osteoarthritis, reduces the risk of cancer, and has been shown to help reverse diabetes and heart damage. Broccoli is best lightly steamed or gently stir-fried; overcooking will neutralize its benefits.

Cabbage: A source of Vitamins K, C, B6, folate, and thiamine. Cabbage is also a source of iodine to support the health of the brain and the nervous system. This vegetable, which is a staple in Chinese kitchens around the world, helps to lower cholesterol and is rich in glucosinolates that are shown to have cancer prevention properties.

Carrot: Raw or cooked, carrots are a rich source of Vitamins A and C, calcium and iron, and the anti-oxidant beta-carotene that gives the vegetable its orange colour. In addition, carrots contain fibre, Vitamins K and E, potassium, folate, manganese, magnesium, zinc, and some phosphorus. Carrots improve our vision, delay aging, help with regulating blood sugar, improve digestion, and help prevent cancer. There is a side note to add: overconsumption of carrots can be toxic so, if you start turning orange, you may want to cut back on your carrot intake!

Cauliflower: The cauliflower is packed with vitamins such as B1, B2, B3,

B5, B6, B9, C and K, as well as being rich in omega 3, fatty acids, fibre, manganese, and potassium. Apart from delivering powerful antioxidants, cauliflower is a healthy source of protein and fibre, it enhances the body's ability to detoxify, reduces the risk of inflammation and the incidence of cancer. Cauliflower is best lightly cooked through a simple sauté.

Spinach: Spinach is widely acknowledged to be rich in vitamins and minerals such as magnesium, iron, copper, calcium, potassium, and zinc. The dark green spinach is packed with anti-oxidants and health-promoting phyto-nutrients. If you're low in iron, spinach helps to make up the deficit. It is an aid in the management of diabetes, and works towards lowering high blood pressure and improving bone health. Spinach is best eaten lightly steamed, quickly boiled or sautéed.

Ginger: Mankind's historic cure-all, ginger is rich in anti-oxidants, vitamins and minerals, and also contains omega-3 and omega-6. Shown to be anti-inflammatory, anti-cancer, anti-nausea, and a powerful anti-oxidant, it greatly boosts the immune system. A versatile root, ginger can be chewed fresh, steamed, boiled in water to make tea, or grated and added to sautéed dishes.

The state in which it is consumed will affect its benefits greatly. Fresh ginger root fights the common cold, coughs, and asthma, while dried ginger root is better against abdominal pain, cold limbs, and rheumatism. If you were to use the fresh root for rheumatism, the condition will worsen but, fresh or dried, it is effective in preventing or stopping vomiting and diarrhea. Large quantities of fresh ginger are not recommended for those with high blood pressure, inflammatory bowel disease, ulcers, or intestinal blockage, and should be used sparingly if you suffer from gallstones. Excessive consumption can cause a person to break out in a rash as an allergic reaction and may also lead to heartburn, bloating, gas, belching, and even some nausea. From ginger root, we'll move on to alkaline-forming fruit and herbs to round up our short list of recommended foods. Remember, some foods are mildly acidic and some are weak acidic foods. Not all acidic foods are tarred with the same brush, but the worst offenders include processed foods, sugar, tomatoes, onions, garlic, dairy, and vinegar.

Apricot: the fruit and the seeds are effective alkaline-forming foods. Packed with iron and protein, apricots are good for quenching thirst and fighting asthma. The seeds from the bitter apricot heal coughs, sore throats, and constipation, as does the sweet apricot seed. But those suffering from asthma should eat only the bitter apricot seed, or the condition will worsen. Laetrile, a naturally occurring substance found in the kernels, has been increasingly promoted to help in cancer treatment. The apricot kernels have been documented to help fight against tumors as far back as 502 AD. The apricot oil has been used as far back as 17th century England to fight swellings, tumors, and ulcers

Peppermint: a herb with healing benefits dating back to ten thousand years in the past, peppermint is commonly used to fight inflammation. It soothes abdominal pain, indigestion, irritable bowels and bloating, and prevents nausea and vomiting. It is a popular healing food for the common colds that are accompanied by headaches, sore throat and thick phlegm. However, if you are suffering a common cold but have a runny nose, cold limbs and diarrhea, peppermint is not that effective. Although it is commonly thought of as an herb or a spice, it is actually cool and pungent, and should not be used daily. Those suffering from anemia or low blood pressure should use only as directed.

"Health is the greatest gift, Contentment is the greatest treasure, Confidence is the greatest friend, Enlightenment is the greatest bliss." -Chinese proverb

FOODS TO ACCELERATE HEALING OF CUTS AND WOUNDS

Skin is the biggest organ in our bodies, and we tend to take it for granted because small nicks heal quickly. However, there are times when there is a deep cut or wound from an accident or from surgery when extra support is required for the connective tissue to regenerate. Connective tissue is different from most other tissues because it is made not so much of cells, but from protein, notably collagen, fibres encased in a unique covering called a fascia. To boost your ability to heal quickly from cuts and wounds, look for foods with these four pivotal nutrients and minerals.

Vitamin C: Vitamin C assists in forming collagen to repair the connective tissue in the blood vessels, cartilage, muscles, and in the bones. Good sources of Vitamin C include fruits such as guava, kiwi, strawberries, and papaya. Vegetables include red and green sweet peppers, Brussels sprouts, broccoli, cauliflower, and sweet potatoes.

Vitamin A: Some of the foods mentioned in the category above will be useful for sourcing Vitamin A because they are rich beta-carotene that is converted into fully active Vitamin A. This vitamin serves many functions. It promotes growth, maintains the immune system, and supports vision. Other Vitamin A rich foods are sweet potatoes, pumpkins, carrots, spinach, turnip greens, and cantaloupe.

Flavonoids: These are a group of pigments that give plants their colour but are compounds that have been discovered to have anti-oxidant properties that are more powerful against a wider range of oxidants than the traditional antioxidants. They help the body detoxify, reduce inflammation, and prevent and reduce damage at the cellular level. Within this grouping, it's the flavonoid called catechin, which is found in great abundance in tea leaves, that is thought to inhibit the growth of cancerous cells. In addition to green, black, and oolong teas, flavonoids are also found in dark coloured berries, bananas, all citrus fruits, parsley, gingko biloba, and cocoa with chocolate content exceeding 70%.

Zinc: This mineral repairs damaged tissues and aids in healing wounds by generating proteins and other genetic material, boosts cell division andcollagen formation, and regenerates tissue, all of which are crucial to wound repair. It boosts the system, develops and activates the T-cells that fight off infection. Zinc is found in vegetables, nuts and seeds such as asparagus, bamboo shoots, Brussels sprouts, okra, potatoes, pumpkin, Swiss chard, lima beans, peas, pine nuts, cashews, pumpkin, and sunflower seeds.

KEEPING YOUR BRAIN HEALTHY

Fernando Gómez-Pinilla, professor of neurosurgery and physiological science in UCLA, describes food as a "pharmaceutical compound that affects the brain".

Studies conducted by him show that the brain is highly susceptible to oxidation damage, so foods that are high in antioxidants protect the brain cells from damage and dysfunction.

Omega-3 fatty acids: These fatty acids support the plasticity of the synapses in the brain that affect critical functions. These include learning and memory, fighting off depression, bipolar disorders, schizophrenia, and attention-deficit disorders. The particularly important omega-3 fatty acid is docosahexaenoic acid or DHA, which reduces oxidative damage, improves synapse plasticity, and is needed in the brain's cell membranes. Omega-3s are found abundantly in walnuts, avocados, flaxseed, chia, and kiwi fruit. Though typically recommended as a desirable source of fatty acids, we take a strong stand against salmon as a source of omega-3s. The oceans are filled with toxins such as mercury, dioxin, and more recently radiation, and seafood is filled with these dangerous elements. In our annals of healing, this leads to mental and neurological disorders such as dementia, Alzheimer's, and multiple sclerosis. It is much safer and healthier to find the fatty acids in nuts and fruit.

Folic Acid: The brain needs sufficient folic acid for its functions, and folate deficiency leads to depression and cognitive impairment. Combining folic acid with other B vitamins has been effective in slowing the rate of age-related decline in cognitive function, and in preventing dementia. Folic acid is found in green leafy vegetables such as spinach, asparagus, romaine, dried or fresh beans and peas, as well as in avocados, beets, broccoli, peanuts, sunflower seeds, honeydew melons, cantaloupes, bananas, raspberries, and grapefruits.

FOODS FOR DETOXIFICATION

In our view, a good detoxification is much more than a spring-cleaning. It's like a good oil change – you take out the gunk and replace it with good, clean nutrients that power the body.

We design tailored and customized detoxification programs that both cleanse and support your system. The concept behind our programs is that it's not enough just to flush out the toxins with a juice cleanse. Instead, you need to simultaneously put back nourishment and support that will revitalize and energize the organs and the immune system.

With that being said, the key organ that is most prone to work overload is the liver. The liver supports almost every organ in the body. It is the second largest organ in the body, and any alcohol or drugs taxes it severely. When that happens, the liver performs less than optimally, leading to an accumulation of toxins that in turn cause chronic illnesses. Natural detoxification foods and herbs are best prescribed after a complete diagnosis to know what is best for your body constitution.

Natural diuretics: Foods that flush the body of toxins are essential to a good detoxification or to counteract the effects of an unhealthy lifestyle. Among natural diuretics are watercress, dandelions in the form of tea, celery, and cabbage, in which is found the antioxidant glutathione to improve the liver's detoxifying function. Be advised that natural diuretics must be used with care; the amount and type to be consumed will depend on your individual body type and constitution.

THE TRUTH ABOUT WATER

The third component to balance our Qi is water.

Water covers 71% of the Earth's surface and is vital to all forms of life. Your body ranges between 50-75% of water as body composition varies according to gender and fitness level, because adipose tissue contains less water than lean tissue. Suffering from fuzzy short-term recall, having problems with mental math or reading small print? Those are signs of dehydration. Be careful in your choice of what you drink. Tap water, sodas, and coffee are all acidic. Our rule is 8x8. We recommend drinking at least eight 8-oz. glasses of water a day to neutralize the acid in the bloodstream for better metabolism and more efficient absorption of nutrients. For those looking for alkaline water, we prefer AquaHydrate, which has a pH of 9+, but only use as directed.

"When you are sick of sickness, you are no longer sick." -Chinese proverb

BE AN EMPOWERED MODERN HEALER

We hope this journey into the healing properties of good nutrition will empower you to make the right choices. Whether it is to give you more energy, get you thinking clearly, accelerate recovery from illnesses, or to age with grace, the choice to eat well and live well rests in your hands. You may find the way ahead difficult and you may need a boost to get you started on the right footing. You may have inexplicable aches, pains, or chronic colds and allergies that just simply refuse to go away. Just changing your diet is not enough to get you on the healing path. Whether you seek preventative care or deep healing, we have the alternative modalities to help you with the healing transformation.

The body is a finely-tuned mechanism. It works until it is out of balance and, even then, it seeks to right itself until the imbalance has buried itself too deeply. Once it does, we are assailed with all forms of diseases and ailments, some too deep to be cured with just nutrition.

As practitioners, we tap into the secrets of our forefathers, into healing practices that have been refined and polished and provided to thousands and thousands of patients through six generations of healers. These are intricate and sophisticated methods of diagnosis, healing, and remedies that are the result of centuries of observation and practice that have withstood the tests of time and the tests of western medicine.

We are deeply immersed in a culture of healing and we drill down to the causes of disease and illness by identifying patterns of disharmony in your body. Our methods are gentle and non-invasive, and we examine not just the visible symptoms, but also take into account the subtle, intangible forces that make up all life. As healers deeply ingrained in a compassionate practice, we examine the physical, mental, emotional, and spiritual aspects because the body, mind, and spirit are inseparable. When you consult with us, you benefit not just from our knowledge and experience, but also from the cumulative wisdom and healing of our medical ancestors.

Martin and Herman are 5th and 6th generation healers steeped in Chinese healing traditions preserved through a lineage that dates back to Shaolin Buddhist principles. As father and son, they run their Toronto-based clinic on a mission to bridge the ancient and modern worlds to take healing to the next level. They seek to bring the body's energies to balance through a holistic and compassionate approach to healing. They customize nutritional plans and draw on modalities such as acupuncture and Tong Ren, a specialized energy therapy, Qi Gong breathing and exercise routines to empower the patient in the healing journey. They are currently co-authoring an upcoming book in response to overwhelming demand from their clients. It will be a thorough look at the beneficial properties, compounds, antioxidants, and micronutrients found in food, and will include ancient breathing and exercise secrets that assist in the healing process. Get more information at http://omaniclinic.com.

The Vegan
Lifestyle Solution

Make the connection between
your diet and your purpose

Dagmar Schoenrock

When I was asked to write a chapter for The Authorities book series, my first thought was, "Me, an authority? I'm a compassionate vegan, not a scientist, not a nutritionist, nor do I have a Ph.D." Nonetheless, I realized that there is no authority outside oneself. I am my own authority on the life experiences that I've had, ones that took me from bison farmer to vegan. This transition was clearly a life lesson, showing me that I need to trust myself — to be my own authority. With this in mind, I am grateful to have the opportunity to share with you some of the facts that helped me return to my true vegan state of being.

Every day, in fact, I'm filled with love and gratitude for the many privileges I've been blessed with. My gratitude list is long and it begins with my parents. Thanks to them, I was raised in a country with many civil liberties, a solid economic base and a peaceful society. This wasn't by accident. I was graced with this life because my parents left their homeland and immigrated to the Canadian prairies for the sake of their children. They wanted us to grow up in a free society and live in peace, safe from the political unrest in Europe. From an early age, I knew and appreciated the value of protecting others, sacrificing for others, and peace.

This awareness played a role in how I lived my life even as a child. I would bring home stray cats and dogs, baby birds that had fallen out of their nests, or turtles trying to cross the road, asking my parents to help me reunite them with their mothers. In school, I brought home bullied classmates until the students intimidating them passed by, and they could safely walk home to their own mothers. In college, I participated in fundraising efforts for various charities to eradicate illnesses or poverty. Later, I became a Big Sister and continued with fundraising for various organizations. When I became a parent, I continued my peaceful efforts by donating to environmental and human rights groups, supporting our local green candidate in the elections, and becoming a Girl Guides leader.

I don't believe this involvement in my community makes me unique; I believe this is what connects me to all of you. Like most people, I have a goal to contribute, in some small way and through some small action, to a free and peaceful society where we can all live in harmony and peace. Regardless of our level of contribution to this cause, we are all connected with the common thread of wanting to make the world a better place. Just think of all of the people you personally know who want to make the world a better place — your parents, your family doctor, the leader of your spiritual and/or religious group, your local humane society, the volunteers in your local community, etc. And now think of all of the organizations around the world whose sole purpose it is to make the world a better place by standing up for social justice, animal rights, human rights, or environmental protection. It's quite exciting, isn't it? All of these people, working and volunteering to make the world a better place, often at a personal sacrifice.

So my question to you is this: If so many individuals and organizations are dedicating their free time, careers, or even lives to making the world a better place, why do we still not live in peace and freedom? It doesn't make sense, does it? Shouldn't this common thread of wanting to make the world a peaceful place lead to common solutions for our global issues? And if the solutions were identified, would you be willing to make the sacrifices necessary to make them happen?

That last question is the hardest one. A good analogy can be taken from the movie The Matrix. In the film, the lead character Neo is given a choice of two pills. The blue pill allows him to go to sleep and wake up the next morning believing whatever he likes. The red pill allows him to see the truth. As Neo's mentor Morpheus says, "You have to see it for yourself. After this, there is no turning back. Remember, all I'm offering is the truth, nothing more."

Would you be willing to take a risk and swallow the red pill that shows you the truth? What if you learned that affecting positive change for global issues relating to social justice, animal rights, human rights, and the environment could be as simple as food choices? By adopting a plant-based, vegan diet, we can have a profound effect in all of these areas. Vegan benefits are felt most immediately in our state of health but extend well beyond into improving the global issues that affect us all. As Will Tuttle, Ph. D., and author of The World Peace Diet states, "Mindful eating is the essential foundation of happiness and peace."

WHAT IS VEGANISM?

To understand the potential global impact of veganism, we should start with the definition of that term. Although the practice of veganism has been noted throughout history, the founder of the Vegan Society, Donald Watson, defined the term "vegan" in 1944 as we understand and use it today. In coining the word, he distinguished vegan beliefs and habits from those of vegetarians. Generally, vegetarians abstain from eating meat, whereas vegans reject meat and animal products in all forms. Not only do they not consume meat, dairy, eggs, or honey, true vegans do not use any clothing, accessories or objects made from an animal.

BODY, MIND, AND SPIRIT

The Body: Improved Physical Health

Before I delve into the far-reaching benefits of a vegan lifestyle, I will begin with the personal advantages it brings to individuals. It's easy to say a new lifestyle improves our body, mind and spirit, but our very nature compels us to seek proof, and rightly so. For years, both the medical and scientific communities have been working to provide data that backs up this claim.

Neal D. Barnard, M.D., renowned physician and president of the Physicians Committee for Responsible Medicine, provides some of the most recent data supporting this claim. Results from his clinical study showed health improved on all fronts for participants with a plant-based diet. According to his research, "People not only slim down, but also see their cholesterol levels plummet and their blood pressure fall. If they have diabetes, it typically improves and sometimes even disappears. Arthritis pains and migraines often vanish, and energy comes racing back. Sluggishness vanishes, and they look and feel radiant."

Those are amazing results, aren't they? The physical benefits of a vegan diet go even further than those addressed by Dr. Barnard. Studies also demonstrate a direct correlation between a meatless diet and a lower body mass index (BMI), which is a typical indicator of healthy weight and lack of fat on the body. The International Journal of Obesity reported a six-year study by scientists at the University of Oxford with 38,000 participants of varied eaters (vegetarians, vegans, meat-eaters and fish-eaters) and found vegans to have the lowest BMI by a significant margin.

This lower BMI translates into healthy weight loss. Eating vegan eliminates most of the unhealthy foods that tend to cause weight issues. Once you adopt a vegan lifestyle, you develop an affinity for new foods, and as your palate changes, so do your cravings. By making a wise choice for your body, you begin to feel more positive.

Another benefit that vegans find as a result of their lifestyle is improved energy levels. More and more professional athletes attest to this, and what better source is there than the people whose very careers depend on their energy and stamina? To name just a few, former Celtics player Robert Parish, famed World Series Champion Hank Aaron and gold medal Olympian Carl Lewis are all major advocates of the vegan lifestyle. Lewis says, "I've found that a person does not need protein from meat to be a successful athlete. In fact, my best year of track competition was the first year I ate a vegan diet. Moreover, by continuing to eat a vegan diet, my weight is under control, I like the way I look. (I know that sounds vain, but all of us want to like the way we look.) I enjoy eating more, and I feel great."

German strongman Patrik Baboumian is another successful career athlete following a vegan diet. At Toronto's 2013 Vegetarian Food Festival, he clearly disproved any belief that to be a strong athletic competitor you must consume quantities of meat when he carried a yoke weighing more than 1200 pounds across the stage.

Outside of maintaining a healthy weight, being vegan improves the body physically in other ways. Healthy skin is dependent on antioxidants like beta-carotene and vitamins A, C and E, which are found predominantly in fruits and vegetables. It follows naturally that vegans will receive an infusion of these as compared to non-vegans. The elimination of dairy plays a role as well. Many dairy-producing cattle are injected with the growth hormone IGF-1, which causes swelling, redness, and clogged pores in humans. Even ailments such as PMS, migraines, and allergies decrease significantly with a vegan lifestyle.

The Mind: Improved Mental Health

In a 2012 issue of Nutrition Journal, Bonnie Beezhold and Carol Johnson reported findings that being vegan definitively improves a person's mood. In their study, participants were divided into three groups: omnivores, fish-eaters and vegetarians. After two weeks, participants completed a "Profile of Mood States" questionnaire and a "Depression Anxiety and Stress Scale" questionnaire. What were the results? The vegetarian group showed significant improvements in their mood scores at the end of the two-week trial. The findings were of no surprise to researchers, who have long known that meat and poultry diets are high in arachidonic acid (omega 6), which is linked to clinical symptoms of depression.

It's important to note, however, that omega 6 is an essential fatty acid, meaning our body does not manufacture it but requires it for good health. To find a balanced omega intake, vegans turn to plant sources instead, such as walnuts, pecans, avocado, flaxseed oil and other plant oils. Not only do these omega sources recover any deficiency that not eating meat may cause, they are also the same sources of vitamins known to improve mood. In other words, you're not only removing dietary items known to cause depression, you're adding foods that have the benefit of improving mood – a double bonus!

The Spirit: Improved Emotional Health

The emotional benefits of a vegan lifestyle are closely tied to the physical benefits. The bottom line is this: if you don't feel well physically, you won't be happy. Constant aches and pains quickly turn good emotional health into general unhappiness. Who among us hasn't had this experience? A lifestyle with good health and nutrition at its core can't help but improve your mood. When you eat well, you feel well.

Veganism also provides an opportunity for us to achieve success. Making the transition is not without challenges, and doing so successfully leads to a sense of pride and self-satisfaction. Our emotional health is better when we have embraced something wholeheartedly, as you do when you properly adhere to a vegan lifestyle. Simply put, it feels good to improve yourself and to do good for animals too.

A new lifestyle means new friends as well: another boost for our emotional health. Having a passion for a cause helps us become more outgoing as we seek to share our knowledge and excitement. A good deed shared by many feels even better than a good deed managed alone.

BEYOND OURSELVES

Now that you know about the personal benefits of veganism, it's time to discuss what to many vegans is even more important: how a vegan lifestyle lets us look beyond ourselves to improve the world. Sound dramatic? It is! Just imagine that a change in your lifestyle can implement change for everyone!

The Environment

"The sixteen hundred dairies in California's Central Valley alone produce more waste than a city of 21 million people — that's more than the populations of London, New York and Chicago combined." — Gene Baur, co-founder and president of Farm Sanctuary.

In a report published by the Food and Agriculture Organization of the United Nations (FAO), we learn that meat production has quadrupled in the past 50 years. Today, farmed animals (animals raised for consumption such as cattle, pigs, chickens, ducks, turkeys, egg-laying hens and dairy cows) outnumber people by more than three to one. Initially, "21 million people," "quadrupled in the past 50 years" and "more than three to one" seem like insurmountable figures, don't they? They certainly don't come across as something to be dealt with in the day-to-day life of average people like us. The truth is, these figures are of great importance to each and every one of us, as they warn us of increased global warming, pollution, water scarcity, deforestation, land degradation, species extinction and world hunger.

Consider, for instance, the relationship between farmed animals and global warming. As most of us know, scientists have been studying the results and effects of global warming's rising temperatures, rising sea levels, melting icecaps and glaciers and shifting ocean currents and weather patterns for years. It's no surprise that they've determined global warming is one of the most serious environmental challenges we're facing. So how is the amount of farmed animals related to global warming? The fact is, farmed animals are responsible for 18 percent of the greenhouse gas emissions that contribute to global warming. Just think about that for a minute. If everyone were to adopt a vegan lifestyle, we would cut emissions by almost a fifth.

Another factor in the correlation between the high farmed-animal count and negative impacts on the environment is the amount of water used to maintain them. The organization People for the Ethical Treatment of Animals (PETA) reports that it takes more than 2,400 gallons of water to produce one pound of meat, while growing one pound of wheat only requires 25 gallons. Not only is animal farming a great drain on natural water supplies, it's a major source of water pollution as a result of the animal waste, antibiotics and hormones, chemicals from tanneries, fertilizers and pesticides and sediments from eroded pastures that are found in water run-off.

Expansion of farmed animal production is also a key element in deforestation. In Latin America, 70 percent of what was once forested land in the region is now used for pastures and feedcrops. Land once valued for creating oxygen, filtering pollutants and stabilizing the global climate has been turned over to the farmed-animal industry. The natural benefits of these forests are lost, and species native to them are rapidly becoming endangered or extinct. Stripping the planet's green spaces is literally affecting the chances of your survival.

Equally concerning is the potential for farmed animal populations to cause world hunger to worsen. As more and more societies become dependent on farmed animals for a significant portion of their diet, the demand for meat is growing too rapidly to keep up with. According to the World Watch Institute, if everyone received 25 percent of their needed daily calories from animal products, only 3.2 billion people would have enough food to eat. Let's suppose that figure were lowered by just 10 percent. In that case, 4.2 billion people would be sustained. That's over 1 billion people more! So just think of what the complete removal of all animal products could do. The entire world population, more than 6.3 billion people, would go to bed every night with a full stomach.

The Animals

According to FAO, more than 60 billion animals are killed every year whether for food or product consumption. This figure is absolutely staggering, and it doesn't even take into consideration the number of animals killed accidentally, whether by farm incident, losing a home to crop cultivation or for mere sport.

In Animal Liberation, author Peter Singer explains the reasoning behind animal rights. He states that the basic principle of equality does not require equal or identical treatment; it requires equal consideration. This is a sentiment shared by many vegans. The question is not whether animals can reason or speak or function at a higher learning level. An inability to state their cause doesn't mean they don't have one. The question, asserts Singer, is whether animals deserve to be free of suffering.

Other proponents of animal rights would point to the selective nature of our diet. Eating a dog would be viewed with disgust in any American home. But a pig? Not an issue. Why is that? In this instance we have two animal species – just two among thousands – that have an equal ability to feel pain, fright, frustration, and contentment. Yet even with their "equal" abilities as higher thinkers, we feel justified in considering one species worthy of our loving homes and one species worthy of being our dinner.

At one time, the term "humane meat" began to take root in the agriculture industry in hopes it would improve relations with animal rights advocates. It meant that eating meat and dairy was justified if the animals were raised in good conditions and not mistreated. That concept, never accepted by vegans, is now beginning to erode with the general population too. Increasingly, reports are published of continued animal cruelty, and secret recordings by nonprofits such as Mercy for Animals are providing the proof. When we see the evidence on video, it is much harder to forget at our next meal how the meat came to be upon our plates. It is also much easier to see the value of a vegan lifestyle beyond its health benefits.

Righting Social Injustices

The social injustice of meat, dairy, egg and honey consumption is a direct result of speciesism: the belief that being human is a valid reason for human animals to have greater rights than non-human animals. To illustrate this point, a vegan will justifiably ask: Isn't raising animals for consumption another form of slavery? Treating a living and responsive creature as an object whose sole purpose is to fulfill our needs…this is slavery in its purest form.

Gary Smith, co-founder of Evolutus, has remarked, "150 years ago, they would've thought you were absurd if you advocated for the end of slavery. 100 years ago, they would have laughed at you for suggesting that women should have the right to vote. Fifty years ago, they would've objected to the idea of African-Americans receiving equal rights under the law. Twenty-five years ago, they called you a pervert if you advocated for gay rights. They laugh at us now for suggesting that animal slavery be ended. Someday they won't be laughing."

What's most striking about this is not the list of victimized and oppressed. Mankind has suffered victimization since the beginning of its history. What's most impressive is that the groups Smith refers to were successful in achieving their goals, however far-reaching they seemed at the time. They advocated their cause with an unwavering commitment to succeed that yielded results once never dreamed possible and were rewarded with magnificent outcomes. In the case of animals, they have no voice to advocate their cause, so it is imperative that we feel compassion towards them. Vegans are the human "voice" of non-human animals. Perhaps Will Tuttle, Ph. D., author of The World Peace Diet, provided the most effective inspiration for dedicating ourselves to the vegan lifestyle when he said, "The light of the infinite spiritual source of all life shines in all creatures. By seeing and recognizing this light in others, we free both them and ourselves. This is love."

Spreading the message

As more and more information comes to light that evidences why a vegan lifestyle has such positive global ramifications, we now turn to sharing that message with others. Every time we turn on our laptop and connect to the Internet, we have the opportunity to educate others on the importance of veganism through various social media sites. We are now able to meet, support, and discuss with people from all over the world instead of being limited to our nearby communities. The Internet provides an opportunity for vegans to stand together through online petitions and fundraising too.

As convenient and effective as the Internet is, let's not forget personal, face-to-face communication. Open a dialogue with a stranger or include a stranger in a conversation you're having with a vegan. Volunteer in a vegan group whose mission is to spread the word. Great strides can be made by working together. Lead by example and model veganism for others. Many people believe they'll have to sacrifice too much of what they love if they become a vegan. Invite guests over and prepare a vegan meal to show them what the food is like, but don't stop there: send the recipes home with them if they're interested. That small effort on your part will go a long way. The small amount of time you save them in searching for a recipe might be enough to encourage them to try out a new vegan lifestyle.

It is important to share the reasons for a vegan lifestyle; it's also critical to use the right means for doing so. In *Why We Love Dogs, Eat Pigs, and*

Wear Cows, social psychologist Dr. Melanie Joy says, "Often, vegan advocates assume that a person's defensiveness is the result of selfishness or apathy, when in fact it is much more likely the result of systematic and intensive social conditioning." With this in mind, approach each person thoughtfully and carefully. Remember, you're asking people to turn their world upside down. Their scepticism is natural. A pushy, demanding, or righteous presentation of facts usually only ensures defensiveness, annoyance, and a pre-determination to not try something new. Using a compassionate, gentle approach will yield greater benefits by far.

LAYING DOWN OUR WEAPON

More than 50 years ago Mahatma Gandhi said, "The most violent weapon on earth is the table fork." Today, science is able to prove the truth in Gandhi's statement. The negative effects of consuming animal products surround us: our forests are being decimated, the climate is increasingly unstable and atrocities against animals are worsening. The good news is that it's not too late to stop the devastation. I said earlier in this chapter that the common thread binding humanity is its desire for harmony and peace.

It was also Gandhi who said, "Be the change you want to see in the world." Each and every one of us has the opportunity to be the change we want to see in the world through the choices we make. I choose to follow in Gandhi's footsteps by living a vegan lifestyle towards harmony and peace. What do you choose? Here, now, is your opportunity. It's as simple as living vegan. If we individually do our part as vegans, then collectively we will have taken massive strides toward achieving our goal for peace. Will you join me in changing the world?

To learn more about a vegan lifestyle, please visit my website at www.MrsGreenjeansPlantsSeeds.com/book, where you can get a free list of hidden animal ingredients in foods.

One Step at a Time

Parents, Educators and Children with Autism share their success stories

Anne-Carol Sharples

We all have aspirations and dreams for our children. Sometimes these expectations begin during our own childhoods as we dream about becoming parents. Sometimes the hopes and dreams do not begin until we look into the eyes of our newborn. No matter when the dream begins, no one dreams of autism. The diagnosis is a sucker-punch that leaves parents reeling and confused. Life quickly becomes complicated with all kinds of well-meant advice from professionals, family and strangers which include everything from medication to diet to the latest new therapy. This chapter does not offer advice on medicines, diet or therapies. The intention of this chapter is to uplift and inspire you. Perhaps you lay awake at night wondering, how I can fight the stigma related to the diagnosis. Maybe you cry, not because of who your child is, but because your child will not fit into the mold society expects. Please sit back and take a moment to learn about the successes of these autistic children and adults. It is with much love and respect that this chapter is dedicated to people on the autism spectrum as well as their families, teachers and caregivers.

SASHA

Sasha met all of her developmental milestones up until 22 months of age. It was then that the gregarious toddler fell silent. The daughter who was stringing two words together saying "What's this?" with inquisitive eyes vanished. Games and activities that Sasha once enjoyed no longer interested her. Eye contact became fleeting and she rarely responded to her name anymore. Sensing red flags, Sasha's parents Marjorie and Ryan began piecing the puzzle together. Shortly after, Sasha was diagnosed with autism. Devastated, but determined to bring back the vivacious child they once knew, the family began a courageous journey that would challenge every aspect of their personal relationships.

Investigating therapies, spending what seemed like hours on the phone and placing Sasha on waitlists left them disconcerted and worn out. Turning to one another for support, they drew upon each other's strengths and continued to map out the next steps in the journey. Together they discussed therapy options, and often reached for the other's hand when either one awoke panic stricken in the middle of the night, worried if they were doing the right thing.

Engaging Sasha in experiences and pulling her out of her shell that she so often retreated into became their undertaking. Sasha began Intensive Behavioral Intervention Therapy (IBI) on a daily basis. Family outings and activities took place every weekend. Rather than shielding Sasha from the world that overwhelmed her, her family wanted her to experience it in positive ways.

Sasha continued IBI until she turned four. It was then that Marjorie and Ryan registered her at the neighborhood school. Beginning kindergarten proved to be very challenging for Sasha and her family. The one-to-one therapy she'd been receiving each weekday was a stark contrast to the room filled with twenty-five boisterous children. IBI Therapy was usually quiet and controlled; the kindergarten classroom was anything but quiet! Sasha was overwhelmed and the first few weeks of school were traumatic for her. As Sasha entered the classroom each day a change would come over her. Her muscles tensed, arms and legs flailed, hands became fists and her jaw clamped shut. Sasha was in protective, fight mode. She was uncommunicative, confused and often distressed, making it impossible to participate in classroom activities. When the other children would sit in circle time and share their stories, she'd become increasingly agitated. Sasha's parents were quite concerned as she collapsed with exhaustion at the dinner table each evening, but they knew her adjustment would take time and vowed to continue taking her to school. What they did not know then, was that school would be the turning point for their daughter.

Marjorie and Ryan decided to use their beloved family outings as a way for Sasha to engage at school. They began to send in pictures of her with short anecdotes written on them. There were pictures of Sasha with her pet bird, at the pumpkin patch, visiting the zoo and opening presents on her birthday. On each of these pictures, Marjorie wrote about each day and what was occurring in the photograph. Over time, Sasha began to respond to these photos when her teacher shared them with her classmates during circle time. Slowly, with support from her teacher, Sasha began to sit for circle time. She'd become very excited when she saw a picture of herself. Sasha's teacher, Mrs. Watson, knew she wanted to share the stories of the pictures herself, so she would have Sasha stand beside her and share her stories through pointing and babbling. Sasha was beginning to communicate at school.

Mrs. Watson played a vital role in Sasha's success at school; for instance, she recognized that Sasha was overwhelmed by the large number of students in the class, so she assigned her a spot right next to her during circle time. She also introduced a visual schedule so that Sasha would know what to expect throughout her day. When there was an unanticipated disruption in her schedule, Mrs. Watson used an "Oops" card to demonstrate the change. Sasha began to communicate with Mrs. Watson by babbling and pointing to the pictures on her schedule. When she was hungry, she pointed to a picture of "snack." She even began to switch her schedule around to her preferred activities and would giggle while proudly showing Mrs. Watson the changes she had made. Sasha grew to love Mrs. Watson; she had a gentle tone of voice and made everyone feel welcome in her classroom. She made school fun for all of her students and her love for teaching shone through her interactions with the students. In addition to utilizing the photographs Sasha's parents sent in, she also recognized Sasha's love for books. Mrs. Watson provided her with a copy of the story she was reading to the class each day. Sasha could hold her book and look at the pictures while Mrs. Watson read aloud to the class. This was a simple yet effective way of keeping her engaged during story time.

Sasha was fortunate to have Mrs. Watson as her Senior Kindergarten teacher the following year. This is the year she began to speak. It began with a word mixed in with gibberish and pointing. It was easy enough to understand, so whoever Sasha was communicating with could model the appropriate language. Soon she began stringing two words together, then two became four so that "blah, blah backpack" became, "I want my backpack."

Sasha is now in first grade and loves school; she reads, writes and talks constantly. The other students adore Sasha because she is persistent, passionate and a joy to be around. She loves to share stories of family outings with her teachers and classmates, with or without photographs.

HENRY

When our son, Henry, was three years old, we were told that he'd never speak or be able to perform simple tasks. We watched, on pins and needles, as the developmental evaluator modeled the activity of stacking three blocks on top of each other and held our breath as she handed the blocks to Henry for him to duplicate what she'd done. Our hearts broke when he was unable to even attempt to stack them. After this evaluation, his father and I were told that Henry would need to be institutionalized. After the shedding of countless tears and multiple late night discussions, we knew that we would not put our son in an institution. We refused to give up hope that we could find a way to help Henry. We enrolled Henry in a school that offered special needs classrooms.

We were fortunate to find a wonderful group of teachers who worked tirelessly to see that Henry was able to function to the best of his ability. After two years in school, with the inclusion of daily therapy, he was able to communicate, albeit in a limited way. Henry never entered a mainstream classroom, but he has achieved multiple successes. The educators and assistants in Henry's special needs classrooms refused to accept the idea of can't. They repudiated the limitations that had been placed on Henry by various doctors and educational evaluators. They only saw what Henry could do and the sky was the limit as far as they were concerned.

Over the years Henry learned how to not only stack blocks, but to tie his shoes and dress himself. He will never hold a job or live by himself, but Henry has made huge strides from what we were originally told he would be able to accomplish. We know that institutionalization would not have been the best choice for Henry as he never would have progressed to the level that he is at today.

ABIGAIL

Here it was again, the dreaded block test. Abigail's grandmother, Eleanor, rolled her eyes as she watched the evaluator hand the blocks to Abigail. She knew Abigail would not stack the blocks or build the bridge the evaluator had shown her. Why are these blocks so important anyway she wondered? Abigail was four years old and had missed most of the developmental milestones. She was not yet speaking coherently; in fact, Abigail had little interest in speaking and seemed unconcerned if her needs were not met. She was absorbed by her own world and took little notice of anything occurring around her. Eleanor wondered if this was because Abigail's mother had abandoned her when she was eighteen months old. She suspected the troubles were compounded by issues in addition to abandonment and was not surprised by the diagnosis of autism. She was surprised when the healthcare professionals told her that Abigail would likely never speak or communicate because she was locked inside her own world. Institutionalization was mentioned, but quickly dismissed by Eleanor. She knew there was more for Abigail and held on to hope that she would find help for Abigail.

As it turned out, help was found during Abigail's first year of school. She started out at age five, a year behind most of the other children in the Junior Kindergarten class. Abigail's teachers and support staff read through the medical and behavioral evaluations and chose a course of action: Abigail was taught just as the other children were taught, with patience, love and repetition. Her teachers did not become frustrated when Abigail stared blankly and did not repeat the sounds they were asking her to make. Instead, they simply tried again the next day. Gradually, Abigail began to come out of her shell, appearing more aware and less self-absorbed. She haltingly began to repeat sounds, then words.

After two years of kindergarten, Abigail was speaking and able to communicate her needs and desires. Her comprehension moved more slowly; it was not until grade three that Abigail began to understand that she should take off her jacket when she felt warm. Her schoolwork moved slowly, as well. Her teachers spent extra time working with her each day and she worked with her grandmother and tutors in the afternoons and throughout summers.

Over the years, Abigail spent countless hours working after school with her tutors and teachers. Her grandmother worked tirelessly to see that Abigail reached her goals. Abigail graduated from high school and is now living on her own in an apartment with two other girls. She even has her dream job working at an amusement park she loved going to as a child.

MARIAH

My name is Mariah and I am twenty-one years old and I have autism. What autism means for me is that I am an excellent painter. I paint better than your average person does. I used to go to school, but now I am finished with school and can paint any time I want. This is very exciting for me because I love to paint; it's my favorite thing to do! My dad takes me and my paintings to art shows where we sell the paintings. My dad always says to do what you love and you will be happy.

MARIAH'S DAD

Mariah struggled with school. She is an excellent reader, but struggles with short-term memory and cannot recall recently taught basic math functions. She was teased often and never understood why the other kids didn't behave as she thought they should. She would often tell the other children what to do, an action that did not win her many friends. She didn't understand the rules of the playground and would push other kids off the swings when she wanted a turn. Her mother and I worried that she'd never be able to hold a job due to her lack of social skills and memory struggles. We wanted more for Mariah. We can provide for her financially, but wanted her life to have quality. We wanted Mariah to be joyful and content.

When she was in her first year of high school, Mariah took an art class and fell in love with painting. She loves the vivid colors and the feel of the paint. Her art teacher recognized that, not only did Mariah have a talent for painting, but that painting was restorative for Mariah. If Mariah was having a rough day at school, her teacher would bring her to the art room where she could calm herself with paint. Her mother and I were stunned at the artwork she brought home. Painting gives Mariah joy. She loves to go to art shows and speak with people about her paintings; she could talk about her paintings for hours! She has felt true success by giving enjoyment to others with her artwork. Since she is able to experience other people's reactions to her paintings, she is inspired to continue working on her craft. Mariah's struggles with interacting with other people evaporate when she speaks of her art. People may not understand Mariah's way of thinking, but they understand her art.

Art is the desire of a man to express himself, to record the reactions of his personality to the world he lives in. Amy Lowell, poet

LILY AND CHARLENE

Charlene will never forget the first day she met Lily. At that time, Lily's only way of communicating was to scream. Lily was four years old, an only child who lived in a low-income apartment with her father. At the time Charlene met her, Lily had received no prior intervention; she was a cautious girl who clung to her father's leg on that day in her apartment. While Lily's father was giving Charlene a snapshot of what the first four years of Lily's life had been like, Lily let it be known that she was displeased with the disruption to her routine. She screamed, climbed the furniture, and removed her clothing in protest. The volume of her screams pierced the air and her father worried that the neighbors would complain, yet again, about the noise. Her father explained that he had been unable to accomplish basics, such as getting Lily to sit in a chair to eat.

The years of struggle, both financial and emotional, wore on his face; he was desperate for help. His spirit was broken, beaten down by the everyday demands of life and compounded by his daughter's needs and his inability to understand her. Charlene desperately wanted to help and felt as though she were carrying a load of bricks as she walked away from their apartment, weighted down by the father's anguish for his daughter.

Charlene went to the school where she was employed as a support worker to speak with the principal about helping Lily. Principal Anderson's son is on the autism spectrum, so he related to the anguish Lily's father was experiencing. Plans were made and Lily began Junior Kindergarten the following week. To say that Lily's first day was exhausting for not only Lily, but also her dad and the staff would be an understatement. The five minute walk from their apartment building to the school took more than half an hour as Lily battled her father every step of the way. Upon arrival at school, it took another fifteen or so minutes for Lily's dad to convince her to enter the building. She made it to the threshold of the classroom and remained there all day long, screaming whenever anyone entered her space or tried to engage her. This continued for several weeks, and throughout that time Charlene persevered by remaining calm and respecting Lily's need for space. By doing this, Charlene gained Lily's trust along with the admiration of the classroom teacher and the staff within the school.

Charlene had a unique way of interacting with Lily; she understood that Lily's behavior was her only way of communicating. She treated Lily with dignity and respect and accepted her where she was. Charlene recognized how difficult school was for Lily and took baby-steps with her, acting as a guide who would remain with Lily until she was ready to go it alone. Over the weeks Lily moved from the threshold of the classroom door to learning how to sit inside the classroom, with Charlene at her side. This was accomplished with patience and kindness, but also with a song. "Row, Row, Row Your Boat" was sung to alert Lily that it was time to enter the classroom and sit down. Lily liked the song and began to request it by holding her hands out and rocking back and forth. Charlene found an old wooden boat and brought it into the classroom so that Lily could sit in the boat and rock it from side to side. This was a motivating experience for Lily since she loved to rock. It is from sitting in the boat that Lily learned how to sit in a chair.

Charlene shared the idea of singing the song with Lily's father. He began singing the song at home to alert Lily that it was time to sit down to eat. Her father was overjoyed when Lily joined him at the table, sat in a chair and shared a meal with him. Charlene was able to accomplish so much with Lily by taking the time to get to know and understand her. It is individuals like Charlene, who have an innate ability to be present and want to help, that make peoples' hearts smile. Lily's father's heart was smiling by the end of her Junior Kindergarten year as he found hope for his daughter's future.

CAITLIN

Mondays are the best. At least Caitlin thinks so because Monday is horseback riding day. Caitlin is fifteen years old and has been diagnosed with autism, in addition to several other health concerns. Caitlin does not have much energy and, as a general rule, does not enjoy exercise. However, she loves all things horse-related; she enthusiastically shows up for her horseback riding lesson and will brush her horse and clean out his stall with gusto. Not every day goes so well. Caitlin struggles when things do not go as she expects and some days Caitlin becomes irritated with her horse and kicks or even punches him out of frustration. Caitlin is working on developing patience, accommodating changes to routine and communicating with her horse without kicking or punching.

Her mother is thrilled with the life lessons, as well as the Hippotherapy Caitlin has received and has shared Caitlin's successes with her special needs classroom teacher, Mrs. McFray. Being quite perceptive, Mrs. McFray decided to explore Caitlin's interest in other animals. She learned that Caitlin has a passion for all animals; therefore, Mrs. McFray incorporated a classroom unit on animals and even obtained a grant to purchase several animals for her classroom. The animals, which include a turtle, a bunny, two guinea pigs and a hedgehog have been a huge hit with all of the students in the special needs classroom.

Caitlin's favorite is the bunny, Mr. Cuddles. She loves to feed him mint and watch him motor his way through the stalk. The students have learned that they cannot hold or pet an animal when they are angry because the animal will become frightened. Prickles, the hedgehog, rolls into a tight ball when she is scared or hears loud noises. Mrs. McFray believes that her students know exactly how Prickles feels. The students can only hold Prickles when they are quiet and calm; they are learning to self-regulate in order to interact with a classroom animal. The classroom pets are treasured by all; therefore the students are highly motivated to regulate their emotions. Because Mrs. McFray took the time to listen to Caitlin's mom, ponder what she heard, and explore options for incorporating animals in her classroom, all of the students have benefited. Mrs. McFray has a deep affection for her students and wants to offer each of them the best learning environment possible.

MILES

Hi, my name is Miles and I'm fourteen years old. I always knew there was something different about me, and it was confirmed when I was seven and told that I have Asperger's Syndrome. Fitting in at school, or anywhere else, has always been difficult for me. I wanted friends, but couldn't figure out how to make them. Things would start out okay, but after a while I noticed that my friends would not be around our usual hangouts. Even worse, when they'd see me they would turn their backs or walk away. I never understood what I'd done wrong. Having friends, then immediately losing them was the hardest part of school for me. The schoolwork was easy-peasy and I probably could've done it with my eyes closed. Recess was a nightmare. At least it was a nightmare until I met Mrs. Wiley and began attending the Program to Assist Social Thinking, aka PAST. I dedicate this story to her. It is due to Mrs. Wiley that I am where I am today.

I began attending PAST one day a week when I was in third grade and I liked it from the start. The best part of PAST is that it is a safe place where we can be ourselves and not worry about anything. You see, all of the kids who attend PAST have autism. And, all of the teachers are super cool and completely understand us. I feel comfortable in my own skin and I can be me when I'm there. Now, that doesn't mean that everything is fun and easy. My teachers challenge me all the time. They know exactly how far to push me and understand when I become frustrated. In fact, they taught me how to control my emotions. Mrs. Wiley, my parents, and my third grade teacher, Mrs. Smyth, would come up with goals I needed to work on at school and at home. So, one of the items my mom really wanted me to learn was how to ask her how her day was and to be genuinely interested in her response. One of the items my teacher wanted me to do was to greet her every morning. Each day I was rated on my performance and scores were tallied up weekly. Once I mastered these goals, other goals were set.

What makes PAST so much fun is that we do super-cool activities, like going rock climbing or to the aquarium that has sea life from around the world. Also, we have a Bearded Dragon in our class! In fact, Eragon, our Bearded Dragon, is such a popular guy, I don't think he is ever in his cage. He has a calming effect on all of us when we are upset. Another activity we do is sit on extremely cool bean bag chairs and do role plays. We also play games to learn about all sorts of barriers that prevent us from being social thinkers. One of my barriers is that I get stuck on what I want to do all of the time. At PAST we have to learn to work as a team and not just do what we want to do. We have a marble jar and each of us puts a marble in the jar when we are being social thinkers. Once the jar is full, we go on an outing; it could be eating at a neighborhood restaurant or checking out the largest indoor reptile zoo. We vote on it and decide. My teacher says we are working, but it feels more like fun than work!

I now realize that my friends used to avoid me as a result of me always wanting things my way. I wanted to be the boss of the whole shebang, from a game of soccer to only talking about what I wanted to talk about. Now I understand that it is important to let other people talk and to listen to them, even if I'm not all that interested. Mrs. Wiley and PAST have taught me how to interact with others and how to have a conversation. Now I know how to start and continue a conversation. PAST has taught me about the perspective of others. I used to think that everyone thought the same way I do. Well, I sure was surprised to find out this isn't so!

Anne Wiley retired from her role as a PAST Teacher in 2014 but continues to volunteer and contribute to the Autism Department at the TCDSB.

A Dream Life for the Asking

Tom Barber

There is an enchanting transformation that occurs during those fleeting moments between sleeping and waking as you emerge out of a deep, relaxed slumber before the demands of the day come tumbling into your conscious world. It is also a magical moment of pure potentiality that contains seeds of inspiration or a solution to that insolvable problem that has hounded you for days. Just as you're about to reach out for that breakthrough thought (the one that teeters on the edge of your consciousness), the alarm clock rings, your smartphone dings a text message alert, your baby cries or your dog bays for food. You lose that thread of inspiration; it's gone as if it never existed.

Have you experienced those moments when you say, "But I just had it in my head, it was *right* there!" only to realize that creativity has tenuously slipped through your fingers?

What if you were able to access this state of pure potentiality as often as you wanted to, when you wanted to? You may require some expert assistance in the beginning to reprogram your beliefs so that you know it is, indeed, possible. However, once you've exercised your "mental muscles" and familiarised your mind and body often enough to get the process fully, you will be able to tap into this infinite source of creativity, inspiration, solutions and possibility at will. What if you could access this untapped power for health, greater happiness and contentment, and for peak performance and success, as if it were "second nature"? Well, you can.

Hypnosis is the technology I use to usher people into deep trance states where they can connect to their inner power. Coined by James Braid, a 19th century Scottish surgeon, the term hypnosis comes from "Hypnos," the Greek god of sleep. You don't fall asleep during hypnosis, however; instead you enter a state of deep, calm relaxation during which you can work directly with your subconscious, that part of your mind that takes care of everything behind the scenes.

Back to that moment in the morning, when you're woken up by the barking of your dogs. From that point on, your conscious mind takes over; it goes through the checklist of what you've got to do during the day, the meetings you've got to attend, the chat you're going to have with your boss or travel plans you're going to make for your next vacation. It seems as if the conscious mind is calling the shots, but actually the subconscious mind is continually doing all the hard work.

It is the subconscious that keeps the heart beating, and that tells your lungs to keep pumping oxygen, which speeds up the movement of your legs as a car is threatening to run you down while you are crossing the street. When you cut yourself, you don't think logically to yourself, "Okay, time for the blood to clot now and the white cells to come fight off infection!" All these seemingly simple, yet intricate reactions are silently and efficiently orchestrated by the powerful subconscious. Think of it as your life's Control Panel.

The pure power of the subconscious is revealed in fleeting moments all the time, even when you're asleep. We're just not always aware it's happening. When you've had a stroke of inspiration, or the genius of an idea, that moment of "divine aha!" leaps out like a Jack-in-the-box, released into your conscious mind. The latter is often met, however, with the vast amounts of data, external stimuli, emotions and physical experiences that are part of your interaction with the world from moment to moment. The trick is to keep the genius intact and to expand its reality within your conscious world. You can learn how to do that too.

The subconscious is the seat of imagination, impulse, creativity and emotion and is also the storehouse of your memories, which means it's one mighty big reservoir. Tapping into it at will and harnessing its power can be truly awesome.

SO WHAT DOES IT ALL MEAN?

What does all this have to do with hypnosis? How can it reveal to us such inner power? Hypnosis takes you to that relaxed state, where your brain frequency literally slows down. Your subconscious mind can then come to the front of the stage as the headline act and revel in the spotlight. In a hypnotic trance state, you remain alert, but you're incredibly focused, just as if you were fully engaged in a really good book or a compelling movie. You switch off external stimuli and are fully engaged in the world of the book or film as if you were right there, in the story.

Hypnosis gives you the key to open the door to the subconscious, access its amazing wealth of information, creativity and resources. It allows you to "anchor" a positive mindset and feelings to be accessed at any point in the future. In this manner, you gain distinct control of your emotions and can manage your mindset for positive behaviour, essentially creating the outcomes you've only ever dreamed of before.

Let's take an example. Let's say you almost drowned when you were a little kid and have since avoided the water. Now an adult, every time you approach the sea, you have a plunging feeling in your stomach. You feel left out on beach holidays because you're afraid of being too close to the water; you don't even dip a toe in the swimming pool. However, you've fallen in love with a marine biologist and you feel that there's something missing if you can't share the love of being in the water with your new partner. Are you always going to stay on the sidelines, or are you going to engage with life so you can have endless fun and build great memories with the love of your life? Which would you choose?

You've been dominated by fear surrounding the bad experience but, with hypnosis, I can take away the sting of the anxiety and terror, as well as any undesirable thoughts that creep into your mind unwillingly at the sight of the ocean. Then, I can help you replace those unhappy memories with a new, more desirable set of emotions and sensory experiences. I can explore with you any feelings of fun, delight and sharing that you've encountered previously in doing something else, like playing football or cooking with friends, and link those feelings with being in the water. By taking these steps, we would together reprogram your mind-body connection so that it reacts positively to swimming and everything associated with it, such as soaking up the warm sun, feeling the breeze, tasting the salt in the water, thriving in the adventure and, ultimately, enjoying more intimate love!

To ensure you can re-access this desirable state, I use a technique called Clenched Fist Auto Anchoring to make sure that these positive emotions are powerfully stored in your body's memory. By anchoring this sensory experience and all its powerfully positive benefits that are meaningful to *you*, it ensures that you can retrieve or spark happy feelings and sensations around water any time you want, in any situation, at will.

Together, through hypnosis, we will have moved you from a previously inhibiting fear to a pleasurable and fearless sense of freedom and adventure. Your whole world will have just changed immeasurably. This is just one example of how well hypnosis works; it is effective in all situations, from helping you pass your driving exam to overcoming your anxiety around public speaking to surmounting weight problems, habits and low-esteem, to finding your life's purpose and creating great success beyond your wildest dreams.

BELIEVE YOU DESERVE MORE, GET MORE

Hypnotherapy is a powerful technology, and it changes lives. The first step forward begins with *you*.

Ask yourself…
- Do you feel that your life could be better lived?
- Do you long to contribute more positively to your family, your friends, your customers and to the world at large?
- Do you feel frustrated because you don't know which direction to take?

- Are you just plain stuck and unwilling to get out of the hole?
- Do you feel there's a vision inside you waiting to be birthed, but you don't know what it is?

The good news is that you'll never have to live another day feeling "less than" or empty, or thinking you're incompetent, unworthy or undeserving. As long as you believe that positive change is possible, that you deserve more than what you're getting right now and that you are capable of great achievements and deeds, positive change is not only possible, it's yours for the taking. What you need now is *the how.*

Hypnosis addresses that "how," that all-important nourishing factor that creates the changes you desire. It's not "if" you can change, but "how" we are going to do this. In my 20 years of experience as a highly qualified psychotherapist using hypnosis and Neuro-Linguistic Programming (NLP), and through my continuing studying and questing, I've found what I believe to be the essential essence that creates the magical moment of true potential where the hypnotic transformation can effortlessly evolve.

The key lies with the ability of one human being to connect with another as well as being deeply attuned to the knowledge and skills inextricably linked to the hypnotic encounter. This is what allows me to connect to the remarkable depth of experience and human-ness of the person who sits by my side. It's about having a true desire to guide you simply through your journey of change, fully believing you can change, even when, right in that moment, your belief is wavering.

Your connection and trust *will* shape and influence the depth of inner journeying, the quality of your therapist's language *will* impact the speed at which you arrive at your desirable state of being, and his or her ultimate belief and faith that change is yours for the taking will impact your ability to access these positive experiences in the future. This I have seen many, many times.

Within myself, I have uncovered the ability to create deep levels of connection with my clients at lightning fast speed, allowing change to happen seamlessly, where extraordinary shifts are open for those who want to achieve, with definitively measurable results. Through my work with many thousands of clients and students, I have harnessed an ability to quickly "feel" where someone is at, to understand how to navigate around their inner terrain and to engage their trust. This ignites their own belief that they can change and really take back control of their futures. I completely believe that change is yours for the taking if you are doing the asking. It is this belief that shines through and creates formidable levels of expectation. When this is in place, the path to change is fully open to the methods and techniques of *how*.

I've been privileged to share amazing transformations as I've delivered conferences and workshops around the world in places such as Eastern Europe, China, Russia and Mexico, all via an interpreter. It's truly phenomenal to experience the depth of the human connection that comes to the fore when words no longer offer a possible means of instant communication, creating a profound and unforgettably moving experience as inner change unfolds before our very eyes.

Such learning has really equipped me to *know* how to move past the words of a story to the deep, true thoughts and feelings of another human being longing for things to change. No two clients are the same, so there's no cookie-cutter approach, but I believe in some fundamentals to embody, some skills that crucially lead the way alongside the "how" for this particular, unique human being with more potential than he or she yet knows. And that's my wonderful job, my life and my inspiration!

My passion for healing others, and my unwavering exploration into my world as my own journey unfolds, places me in the unique position of travelling the path that will need to be walked for this journey of life to evolve further for you too. I've climbed the mountain before, and I know the track well, so I can guide the people I work with from where they are now to where they want to be. And, if they aren't sure about where that is, I can help them locate just what that destination point is too.

My decision to become a therapist fanned an inner flame, which I hadn't known existed, to learn the art of helping others and changing lives. As I engaged in helping others, I found that I tapped into another joy, learning the depths of myself, discovering my inner undiscovered dimensions, becoming freer and more engaged with life and my healing practices. And so the journey continues to unfold.

LIVING A LIFE TO BE PROUD OF

Those are some of the benefits I would like to pass on to you. You see, there is so much that we can do ... and so much that you can do too. You can learn to self-hypnotise for those times when you have no access to a trained therapist, so you can harness your tremendous personal power and live a life of which you are proud.

You might be surprised to discover that you *already* self-hypnotise. We all do. Driving to work and being oblivious of your journey, watching TV and losing track of the plot, finding yourself daydreaming out of the office window. These are all examples of drifting into a state of hypnosis. Imagine learning what you can do with that!

Think about the customs that sports teams go through before a big game – the pre-game rituals and the pep talks that are meant to pump up the team and strike fear in the hearts of the opponents.

In the formidable game of rugby, my all-time passion, the New Zealand All Blacks like to take the temperature up a notch and intimidate the competition by performing the Haka, the traditional Maori dance. It involves loud war cries, heavy pounding of feet, stylised gestures of violence, fierce facial expressions with hanging tongues and glowering stares, all barely feet away from the competing team. Yet, the purpose is not just to frighten off the opposing players; the gestures and stomping are a means of "hypnotising" themselves into states where they are strong, fierce and powerful. It is a means by which they tap into the legendary courage of the Maori warriors of old.

So, a dream life is yours for the asking. If you believe you can have an expanded life with more creativity, more accomplishments, more freedom and more passion, if you believe you can be more aligned, the "how" is right there in your hands. It really is within your reach and your grasp. I invite you to walk the path with me, and would be honoured to be your companion in growth.

Once Tom Barber discovered hypnotherapy, he found himself reinvigorated and re-engaged with life, soon desiring to help others as he was himself helped. He has become a leading Hypnotherapist and Psychotherapist helping people to make changes they so desperately want and can have through hypnosis.

Tom is an international instructor and in-demand Speaker, and is the award winning author of *The Book on Back Pain: The Ultimate Guide to Permanent Relief*, *The Change Sequence*, and Co-author of *Thinking Therapeutically: Hypnotic Skills and Strategies Explored*. Additionally, he is a Director at Contemporary College of Therapeutic Studies UK, where he trains others also wanting to embark on an enriching and fulfilling career in making a difference to others' lives, whilst also co-ordinating SelfHelpSchool™, which provides Self Help through education for the public. Tom, who is known as 'The Changeologist', consults 'leading lights' in the arenas of sport, art and music, as well as the corporate world, all who are committed to inspirational change and growth strategies using the power of the mind. You can contact Tom at Change@TomBarber.co.uk

Declutter Your Mind for Success

Erin Muldoon Stetson

"My baggage", "your baggage", "his baggage" —phrases thrown around in casual conversation as much as an actual suitcase is thrown around by handlers at an airport. What does it mean when we talk about our "baggage?" After all, we're not actually referring to that matching set of luggage your mother bought you after college, are we? No, we are talking about the emotional and life experience "stuff" you pick up along the way; the stuff that weighs you down and makes the inside of your head hurt.

When we take a trip, our baggage literally gets heavier and messier with each souvenir we add. And, if you're like me, you can't wait to unpack and put the dirty laundry in the wash where it belongs. Similarly, in life every experience comes with emotional as well as physical stuff. Unfortunately, not all of it is as pleasurable as the mementos from vacation. Plus, when unpacking, most of us take a look at what comes out of the suitcase so we can put it where it belongs.

But, when it comes to emotional baggage, people tend to stuff it away without really looking at it. What they are doing is filling up the emotional equivalent of a classic, overstuffed closet; the one where, when you open the door, a thousand things come crashing down on your head. The one where you don't open the door except maybe a couple inches now and then to stuff more things into the dark, scary closet.

On an emotional level, that stuffing is doing you no good at all. In fact, all that clutter is not relegated to your subconscious mind. It affects all parts of your mind, as well as your body and spirit. It causes pain, disease and emotional issues. It can block you in countless ways—from achieving your potential, living authentically and manifesting abundance in your life.

Why is your mind so cluttered in the first place? It's because you've been "collecting" experiences, memories and feelings for a lifetime. Even in the womb, there may have been alarming and confusing experiences. If you had a difficult birth, or traumatic first few moments of life, the imprint of those experiences is still with you. To add insult to injury, as a baby, you may have often struggled to be understood or to have your needs met while your bumbling care givers tried to figure out if you were hungry, sleepy or needed a diaper change. How frustrating that must have been. Those early experiences went into your collection.

Think about the clutter you have collected. I suggest that, as you read this, you jot down the thoughts that pop into your head. No doubt you will start to think of your own personal clutter that is stuffed inside you somewhere. Your notes will help you when you decide to clear that clutter out. Remember, you need to look at all of it squarely before you can put it away for good.

The collection of emotional clutter goes on throughout your life. In the toddler years, you stumble and fall (literally), and struggle to communicate only to be utterly misunderstood. Then, as a teen, you stumble figuratively as you try to find your way, and still find communication difficult as your values change in relation to those of parents, teachers or even your peers.

Think about it:

- A humiliating experience in class when a teacher scolded you in front of everyone.

- Someone you had a crush on treated you with contempt.

- A vicious, behind-the-back bullying campaign waged by an alleged "friend."

- A time when you were unkind or ungrateful to someone who didn't deserve it.

- The day you walked out of a store with a pack of gum you didn't pay for.

Each of these experiences is jarring. Every single one of them can disrupt the energy system in your body and mind. It's no wonder you feel so overwhelmed with the clutter.

I vividly remember something that happened when I was 12 years old. I received a scathing note from one of my "best friends" who happened to live across the street. It was poetic in its poignancy. "Erin, you think you're hot shit on a silver platter, but really you're just cold diarrhea on a paper plate!" Wow. That hurt. It's funny now —I mean really funny — and I'm so impressed with the verbiage. But at the time, I cried big tears —the kind of tears that I thought might never stop gushing. I had to re-think my whole persona. Did I really think that I was "hot shit?" And was I actually "just cold diarrhea?" I collected the anger, the sadness and the insecurity of that moment and buried it all in my mind, heart and body.

For the record, I'm not saying that any of the experiences I'm mentioning were bad, or good, for that matter. Nor am I saying that my friend in the "hot shit" story was wrong for writing that note. What I am saying is that our experiences stay with us, in one form or another, and often create disruptions in our energy systems.

Have you been able to jot down a few notes about memories of your own that may have stayed with you and created disruptions in your own life? Job struggles, relationship or parenting challenges, heartache, loss, trauma—the little things and the big things that may be stuffed away, buried, doing some damage unbeknownst to you.

All of these things go into your collection. Don't judge them. Don't judge yourself. Simply write down a "title" for the memory. We'll address it later and possibly let go of it with ease. You won't lose the memory, but merely the negative charge that is connected to it.

Now that you have started to examine your impressive collection, you can understand how it has grown exponentially over your lifetime. You can imagine how your mind has gotten cluttered. It's no wonder so many people feel weighed down, bottled up, distracted and even confused at times.

It is possible to declutter your mind if you have the proper tools. There is a process you can use to fix the effects of that build-up.

Pat yourself on the back for beginning this journey. It's going to be fun!

TAPPING

Tapping is based on Emotional Freedom Techniques (EFT). It is a relatively new discovery that has provided thousands with relief from pain, disease and emotional issues. It can alleviate the most common matters (fear of public speaking) to the most extreme (chronic debilitating back pain), and a wide array of "stuff" in between. Basically, tapping is mind/body healing. It is a combination of ancient Chinese knowledge and modern psychology.

Tapping produces a relaxation response in your body and mind and creates an emotional contentment in the present moment. It is wonderfully simple and effective, and it is accomplished by stimulating well established energy meridian points on your body.

"How do you do that?"

You do that by tapping on particular points with your fingertips while focusing on the issue at hand.

"Really?" "It's not more complicated than that?"

Yes, really. And no, it's not more complicated than that. Plus, the process is easy to memorize, and portable—you can do it anywhere. You only need your hands and your mind.

It is my goal to make this real healing easy and accessible to you. For the entrepreneur feeling overwhelmed, or the person who has dreams of starting a business but is blocked by fear, these techniques can help create such fundamental shifts that walls tumble and doors open. The healing path of body, mind and spirit lies ahead.

So how does tapping differ, say, from other energy healing modalities such as acupuncture? By focusing on the mind-body connection, EFT tapping harnesses the power of the mind and combines it with the body's energy to propel healing to a level that could not otherwise be achieved. The techniques essentially bring a psychotherapeutic element to the energy meridians long familiar to alternative healers.

The power of thought and its effects on our well-being are no longer considered theoretical. The evidence is piling up. So let's declutter your mind so that your thoughts no longer sabotage you but can have the impact you want them to!

EFT TAPPING IN ACTION

Let's look at a particular, very real scenario that will be familiar to many. I like to call it the fear of public writing. Now, we could also address the fear of public speaking or something else but, given the fact that I overcame my fear of public writing to write this chapter, it seems an apropos example. Additionally, the fear of public writing can be a huge deal for an entrepreneur, especially when you are expected to publish a blog, post on Facebook and update your website on a regular basis.

EFT tapping has the unique ability to handle your fears and turn them into calm cool action. Whether you feel paralyzed at the thought of doing an activity like writing, or are shy about sharing what you've already written, EFT tapping can help put those fears in check.

For example, have you hesitated to write a book because of your anxiety about the fact that the dreaded written word can never be erased? It will be "out there" speaking for you, for all time. If you are like I was, that thought paralyzes you. But here I am, writing this. And enjoying it, I might add. How am I able to face my fears so courageously?

As I mentioned above, the answer is quite simple and incredibly revolutionary. I can't wait to share this fabulous secret with you. Tap along with me. You won't be sorry. Then we can high five on the other side of this silly fear that's holding you back from your greatness.

EFT IN A NUTSHELL

The body contains a network of energy points and energy channels — actual locations that can be accessed through tapping. In addition to the physical act of tapping on these specific points, EFT involves the use of words. The power of words, of language, to channel and manifest intention is hardly in question any more. So with EFT, you will use words first to acknowledge the details of the negative — the big pieces of junk cluttering your mind.

Looking at them and facing them is the first step to releasing the junk you've been shoving into your suitcase for so long. Finally, positive language is used to manifest what you want to bring into your life after you've released the unwanted clutter through tapping.

So, let's return to our hypothetical case of a person (maybe you) who is afraid to write. This fear is getting in the way of your business, your success and your ability to create abundance in your life. Below are the simple steps that I would walk you through if you were this hypothetical person. In no time, you would be writing and publishing.

STEP 1

Close your eyes and think about what is holding you back from writing and publishing that book or updating your blog. Once you have something specific in mind, give it a number on a scale of 0-10, ten being the most intense. If you have many things running through your mind, write them down and start with the one specific issue that has the highest intensity. Think of it as the biggest piece of junk in that closet—the one that might actually knock you out if it fell on your head. Give that piece of junk a "title"—you don't need to write down the whole sordid history or explanation of the issue, just its title. The number you assign to that issue is extremely important. It allows you to compare how you feel before and after tapping.

For example, you may be thinking: "What if my ex reads this and thinks, 'what the %&*# is she writing about? Why was I ever with that chick? What a weirdo!'" Or perhaps you are thinking, "No one who reads this will ever want to talk to me, meet me or hire me. I'll be ruined."

Your title for this piece of mental debris might be: Fear of Rejection. Maybe it earns a level of 8, 9 or even 10, depending on how paralyzing it is. (You insert whichever number makes sense for how you feel in the present moment.)

STEP 2

Tap continuously with your fingers on each of the following spots while repeating the corresponding phrases out loud. (If you think a diagram might be helpful, please visit http://taponit.com.)

Karate Chop Spot (this is the place on the side of your hand you would use if you were to use a karate chop to break a piece of wood): Tap continuously with four fingers on that spot while saying the following phrase three times aloud: "Even though I am afraid of being judged and rejected [insert here: by my ex or by future clients] for what I write, I'm still a really good person."

- **Eyebrow point** (this is the beginning of your eyebrow closest to your nose): Tap continuously with two fingers at that spot and repeat the following phrase: "I'm afraid that my [ex or future client] is going to judge me and my writing in a negative way."

- **Side of eye** (this is the bone bordering the outside corner of your eye): Tap continuously with two fingers on that spot and repeat the following phrase: "What if my [ex or future client] reads what I wrote and thinks I'm a terrible writer?"

- **Under the eye** (about 1/2 inch below the eye on the bone): Tap continuously with two fingers, saying: "I'm nervous to put myself out there. I will be laughed at."

- **Under the nose** (this is the philtrum: the small indentation between the bottom of your nose and the top of your upper lip): Tap continuously with two fingers on that spot while you say: "I'm afraid that someone [my ex or a judgmental future client] is going to read my writing if I put it out there."

- **Chin** (the spot inside the indentation midway between the bottom of your chin and your lower lip): Tap continuously with two fingers on that spot and say: "I'm not sure if I can handle the embarrassment of having my writing judged by [my ex, a future client] or anyone else for that matter."

- **Collarbone**: Tap continuously with four fingers along your collarbone towards your breast bone. Say these words: "I'm not ready to have my thoughts and ideas critiqued and ridiculed."

- **Under arm** (four inches below your armpit, on the side of your body): Tap continuously with four fingers: "I'm nervous that [my ex or a future client] will read what I'm writing and make fun of me."

- **Crown of head**: Tap continuously with all five fingers in a circular motion on the top of your head: "I'm afraid that [my ex or anyone] is going to read my writing and laugh at me."

- **Eyebrow point**: "I'm okay now."

- **Side of eye**: "I can relax now."

- **Under the eye**: "I am calm and relaxed."

- **Under the nose**: "My confidence is growing."

- **Chin**: "I am feeling more and more confident about my writing."

- **Collarbone**: "I am excited to write an awesome [book, article, blog]."

- **Under arm**: "I can't wait to write my [book, article, blog]."

- **Top of head**: "I'm ready to write and publish an amazing [book, article, blog]."

When you are done, take a deep breath and hold it. Then let it out in a slow, smooth exhalation.

STEP 3

After completing the tapping and repetitions, reassess the intensity of your feelings about the topic (in this case, public writing), using the scale you used originally, from 0 to 10, with ten being the strongest. Write down your response, the number and something about how you feel. Comment about whether there were any qualitative changes to the way you view or feel about the topic. If your number is still high, then repeat the process.

Be clear in acknowledging any change. For example, "After tapping, my fear of rejection and judgment regarding my writing from [my ex or future clients] is at about a level two, down significantly from my previous level of eight."

The three steps outlined above are how you use EFT to overcome your fear of public writing. You can use the same format to cope with other issues that are holding you back. The phrases that you use in your repetitions during tapping will vary according to what you are trying to release. Here are some examples:

- **Karate Chop Spot**: "Even though I'm afraid that my family will disown me because what I want to write about is too off the grid for them, I have confidence and love. I forgive them for their potential judgments." Repeat three times.

- **Karate Chop Spot**: "Even though I fear that my ideas will change one day, and what I write will be 'out there' forever, reminding me of how foolish I was, I deeply and completely love and accept myself."

- **Karate Chop Spot**: "Even though my writing isn't perfect, it's a work in progress that never seems to end. I am whole, and complete, and fabulous just as I am right now, and so is my writing."

- **Karate Chop Spot**: "Even though I feel as if I don't have time to write, I am willing to make changes in my life because I deeply and completely love and accept myself."

The intended and very real outcome of EFT tapping in this circumstance is increased self-confidence. Whether it is your writing or something else that is standing in your way, your confidence will grow exponentially the more you tap. You will laugh at your previous fears. To use our example of fearing the reaction of your ex, once you have utilized EFT tapping, you might assume that, should he read your writing, he'll wonder how he ever let someone like you get away!

Our fears about what might happen are often times more intense than any actual, potential outcome. Tapping creates equilibrium between that fear and what is real. It will allow you to gain a calm, cool perspective regarding the debris that was weighing you down by cluttering up your suitcase or your closet –in other words, your mind!

Decluttering your mind through EFT tapping applies to literally any aspect of your life. It can help you find fulfillment, success, and enjoyment in any arena: relationships, money, body image, health etc. Starting with identifying what is holding you back, seeing it for what it is and then releasing it, you ultimately replace it with something positive that will help you move forward.

The things that are holding you back are all that junk we talked about earlier: Fears or objections (the "I can't" mentality), obstacles — perceived or real (time, logistics) — and ultimately your "story" – the belief system that holds you where you are instead of helping you get to where you want to be.

The process that works for your mind can also be used to declutter your body. There is a holistic connection between and among mind, body and spirit, which means that detoxing one will help you connect with the others to live your best life.

In using EFT techniques for the spirit, you will address matters of perspective, outlook and attitude. The law of attraction is essentially at work every time you succumb to fear or, conversely, feel optimistic. When you fear an outcome and fixate on that fear, you are focusing on what is essentially a belief system based on fear. Your mind, as well as your actions, reflects that belief system and you will manifest the very things you are afraid of.

When you can tap on and release the fear, you can recreate a belief system based on positive emotions, optimism and confidence. You become that person and your every action reflects those new beliefs.

So what does this mean for you? It means that EFT tapping can bring you more comfort, love and enjoyment in life. It can help you rid yourself of the heavy baggage and clutter that get in the way of being your most successful self.

To learn more about the benefits of tapping, please visit http://taponit.com.

Awakening Your Healer Within

The Miracle of You
PHILIP YOUNG

In this book you will glean information from "authorities" who offer mind-expanding ideas and concepts that will benefit your entire life and wellbeing. After countless hours of extensive study, thousands of client sessions, and twenty-five years experience, I am excited to be an authority. In my case, the particular subject of expertise is energetic healing and, like the other authorities in this book, I am pleased to share some of this information and knowledge with you. When learned and understood correctly, energetic healing has the ability to uplift, enlighten, and heal either you or a loved one.

To begin, we must define energetic healing. This is a metaphysical healing that takes place beyond the limits and assumptions of physical science known today. In reading this, you will learn how your inner, non-physical energy affects your health and wellbeing, and how this non-physical energy can be harnessed to assist you, sometimes in miraculous ways.

Today, most people see good health as something that is outside of their control, something that they have to fight to maintain. Health is also usually seen as that which is administered to them by outside medical experts and specialists, but there is another approach. What would it be like if, instead of seeking immediate traditional medical assistance, we embraced and recognized the body's own infinite wisdom? Could we then make changes from within? As people are able to open their minds to it, the answer to this question is most emphatically yes. All the wise and experienced physicians I've met with agree that, even with the scientific knowledge that has been gained over the years, we still know very, very little about the complexities of the human body. We are just beginning to scratch the surface of the miracle that we are.

The point of mentioning how little we know is to emphasize that there is another way of being, a way that truly 'does no harm' and is ultimately within your own control and power. If chosen, this is a path that leads to a radiant, healthier, and happier life that will help fill you with greater joy and wonder than ever before experienced.

Let's start with history. In ancient times it was understood that the natural state of human beings was one of vibrant health, and that this vibrant health came from the Self within. As science progressed, facts and data began to take precedence and this inherent knowledge was lost, buried, changed, or distorted. Now, millennia later, these truths are slowly being rediscovered.

I'd like to suggest that the secret of your entire health lies within you, and it is something that you can control with intention. It is something to be conscious of and to take responsibility for. This is a concept seldom taught or understood, which is especially regrettable because it takes so little commitment and discipline. In much the same way as other daily habits become routine, such as brushing your teeth, taking control of your health can be just that easy.

Many people regard themselves as victims or survivors of a disease (dis-ease), and this attitude has been encouraged in various ways in our society. It is a viewpoint that diminishes the Self and gives power to others. As you begin to consider yourself empowered as an active director of your own health, you engage your mind, spirit and body with intent, allowing miraculous changes to occur.

Every moment of every day, millions of cells are being created perfectly within your lungs, your organs, and your blood. All this takes place at the will of non-physical energy and is without any conscious effort on your part. It occurs simply by your inherent desire and intent. This is a monumental clue to the Truth and the beginning of realizing that you already are a miracle! This non-physical energy fills and actually enlivens your cells, tissues, and even your DNA. In fact, it permeates your entire being. Without being too esoteric, think of it as a 'Life Force', one that ultimately gives you Life and also determines your level of health and wellbeing. In circumstances when your health may not be currently optimal, this energy may have been compromised in some way. However, with help, application and some minimal training, it can be redirected to once again be a positive and beneficial resource for your body.

The dilemma that we have in our limited and often blinkered western way of looking at the world is that this non-physical energy has yet to be measured by material instruments. Society as a whole believes that, if something can't be measured, it cannot be. This line of reasoning actually mimics that of well-meaning priests from medieval times, who might have rigorously dismissed the concept of radio waves simply because they did not have the means to measure them at the time. That way of thinking is archaic. Non-physical energies can be perceived by those who are trained and considered to be attuned, open, and intuitively gifted. Moreover, the effects of these energies can be seen and experienced by all, whether or not we are aware of them.

For many years I have had the good fortune to help people experience healings that have been described as miraculous and even impossible. The people who have experienced healing have been able to reach a certain place within them of greater possibility. The process felt so natural, gentle, and effortless for them that they were often not even consciously aware of it taking place. In much the same way that you can use a magnifying glass to ignite kindling or paper, with my assistance people are able to reach a place of perfect health, a place Within that they ordinarily could not reach on their own.

So, how on earth do you reach the place Within that is already perfect? It is similar to tuning in to a radio station. In this case, however, you are tuning in to a subtle part of your Self. Continuing the radio metaphor, you may well experience some static, but if you persist you are able to tune in to that perfect part of you. As you invite the energy to come forth, hold a strong and consistent intent. Don't give up. When people struggle with this, occasionally they'll recall how they were when they were little children: carefree, happy, and hopefully in perfect health. A child's mind is filled with the exact joyfulness, openness and trust you are seeking. By holding onto these memories, the process may be easier.

To tune in to this station, it is also important to maintain a conscious feeling of gratitude for your perfect health in this very moment, regardless of present outward appearances. It's also important to suspend the activities of the intellect and ego and to control the mind chatter. You must move gently and in a state of deep relaxation through your feeling Self and through your loving Heart. By allowing yourself to maintain this thankfulness and gratitude for the miracle that you are, you can continue to fine tune this channel of perfection.

Because the process is unfamiliar, it can seem difficult at first. Most people find it far easier to begin with my help, and they always have beneficial results when they do. This occurs simply by my being fully Present with individuals in each visit with them. I speak with and listen to each person with patience and compassion. Using the vibration of my voice, and the heat and healing touch of my hands both on and around my clients' bodies, I'm able to help them find that place of perfection that's Within.

Over the years, I have found that there are always emotional hurts and concerns (real or imagined) that affect the wellbeing of the individual. Often, there are few if any people who have the time, patience, or compassion, and who are willing to listen to these concerns, much less respond in a supportive and loving way. Many doctors and specialists I meet sadly agree that they only have a few minutes to spend with each patient. Seldom do they learn much about the individual's hopes, past, fears, loves, concerns, personalities, relationships or families. So for them, if that were the case, it just wouldn't be possible to determine how non-physical energies may be of help to those in need.

When I meet clients in need of non-physical healing I allow the vibration of unconditional Love and highest intention to come forth. These energies can be felt as heat in my hands. Sometimes people actually think I have electric heating pads placed on their body. My own body becomes very warm, even hot, as these non-physical energies flow. It is a process of surrendering, of trusting without any ego whatsoever. Something much, much greater is present and in control. Usually this occurs for about an hour and then the energies stop, as the individual is complete. It is much the same way as we stop pouring water into a glass when it is full. No more can be added for the time being.

I feel most blessed to share these deep, sacred insights into the world of each individual. It allows for another aspect of their health, wellbeing and hope to blossom forth and then they feel better. True healing has to consider the totality of the person. It's a matter of body, mind, and spirit.

The following pages chronicle a few of the positive results I've obtained during my many years of practice. These anecdotal accounts demonstrate how real people have experienced wonderful results during healing sessions. Remember, if one man, woman, or child can do it, then so can another! Perhaps you are seeking a remedy at a time when other choices seem dim. If so, it could be that I might be able to help you or a loved one in some way. Whatever the reason, our Hearts and minds have crossed here for a sacred reason. I do hope that you enjoy the material on these pages and that you are inspired to implement the ideas for yourself, or perhaps to share them with others. Within the sanctity and authority of your own Self, take Heart, remain hopeful, and have faith that another way is surely at hand.

BREAST CANCER

"Your breasts are all clear."

Many years ago a dear and beloved friend called one day to say she had breast cancer. Little did I know then that her journey would help me embark on my own journey to becoming a healer.

Trish had been diagnosed with breast cancer and she was dreading the usual medical approach of "cut, poison, and burn" that still today seems to be the one size fits all medical standard. She had been endeavoring to learn as much as possible about her disease, including various alternative ways to treat her condition. She was fearful of chemotherapy's associated toxicity and the side effects that she knew would be so debilitating for her long-term health and wellness. She was open to another approach that was not harmful to her.

After many years of my own esoteric studies and interests, I was now faced with the stark reality of speaking my truth and endeavoring to do something for her or saying nothing while still trying to be supportive. Many of us have often found ourselves in similar situations. It's a matter of walking the talk vs. talking the talk.

I asked Trish if she was willing to try some healing after she had a lumpectomy. She answered yes and was, in fact, willing to try anything that might help. One day we sat down on her cottage lakefront and, to the bemusement of her husband and my wife, began to try a healing process I had read about. I felt certain and hopeful that I could really help her. That day, for about an hour we held the first of several such sessions, not really knowing what to expect, but highly desirous of a good outcome. Although these were just early steps at the time, nonetheless the good outcome arrived! Her breast cancer disappeared completely and to this day, over 20 years later, her breasts are cancer free!

LIFE SENTENCE

"We can't understand it. The tumors are gone."

Several months later I received a phone call from Jillian, a woman referred to me by Trish. Jillian had cancer throughout her body and had been diagnosed as only having a month or two to live. She was told to go home and get her affairs in order. We arranged to meet at her home and we spoke at length about what was going on in her life.

For the first five weeks we gently dealt with some personal issues that she had experienced. On each visit as I spoke with her I laid my hands upon her as she went into a deep guided relaxation. She returned to the hospital for follow up scans and tests, much to the amazement (and even anger, she said) of her medical doctors, as she had defied their diagnosis. Her tumors were either shrinking or had disappeared completely! Over the next several months she and I continued her healing sessions to the point where all tumors were completely gone.

I continued to see Jillian occasionally for over a two-year period. Years later, she eventually passed, but her life and vitality had been extended so much to the everlasting joy of her family, friends and loved ones.

COMA

"Your daughter is going to be in a permanent vegetative state. We are sorry, but there is no hope."

I happened to meet Rita by chance in an office where she was working. Rita told me her daughter Katrina had been struck by a car and had been thrown 70 feet. She had severe head trauma and had been in a coma for several weeks and, at this point, it was expected by the doctors that she would be in a permanent vegetative condition. There was nothing more they could do for her.

When I was a little boy I experienced head trauma and have always felt a deep sense of compassion and empathy for those who have head injuries.

When Rita told me about Katrina, I knew that I had to see her. Out of the blue, I asked Rita if she would be open to that and she said yes.

The next day, walking down the corridors of the hospital, part of me was asking what in the world I was doing there. Part of me wanted to get out of there before I made a complete fool of myself. And yet, another part of me was serene, sure, and calm. I felt like something was guiding me.

Rita was already in Katrina's room and we exchanged a few words. The doctors would not know what I'd be doing, but a couple of the nurses had been informed so that we would not be disturbed quite so much. Seeing Katrina so unresponsive on her bed was quite unsettling. What was I going to say to her? How could this possibly work without a verbal exchange? Without any feedback? With no clues from the eyes? Then I felt a still, calm knowing within me that became my guide. I moved the bed out from the wall, leaned over, and put my hands gently on first Katrina's head, then arm, then hand. Her mom simply looked on, accepting. After about 45 minutes, the healing session seemed to be complete. I really didn't know what to expect. This was new territory for me.

A day later, Rita phoned me to tell me that Katrina had moved her thumb and that the doctors had said this was a reflex. I replied that this is exactly the type of reflex we wanted! A few days later I went back to the hospital and repeated the session, gently touching her arm, her heart, as well as her head. Rita phoned again with good news; this time that Katrina had moved her arm. When I checked my messages a couple of days later I heard one from Rita. Katrina had spoken! I was so overjoyed to hear that and tears ran down my face. It was Christmas Day – what a gift! I saw Katrina several more times and I'm so thrilled that she made a full and quite miraculous recovery.

BRAIN BLOOD VESSEL PROBLEMS (AVM)

"I could drop dead at any moment."

Len was recommended by a friend after he was told by the medical specialists that he had a very serious malformation in the thalamus of his brain. The condition is called an arterio-venous malformation or AVM. There was a weakening in the walls of the blood vessels feeding this very intricate and important region of the brain and he was enduring terrible headaches and some numbness in his extremities. His doctors explained that the medical treatment for such a condition was gamma knife brain surgery. If he survived at all, he could have many cognitive deficits. If he did nothing, he left himself at risk of the malformation erupting and of inevitable sudden death. The odds were against him.

I was his last resort and our first meeting was brief. He was short on time and clearly short on inclination to believe in non-physical healing. He told me that he also had tendonitis from playing golf and wondered if I could do something for that, too. Before long he was soon on the massage table in a deep sleep-like state.

I thought things had gone well and after an hour brought him back. He said he felt unusually relaxed, yet he also seemed to be skeptical as to what he had just experienced. Not surprising for such a practical left brain thinking, alpha male. Still, he was very gracious and we said our farewells.

Sometimes, clients will call me soon after our sessions to let me know their good news. I hadn't heard from Len for several weeks and I was beginning to think that perhaps things had not gone so well for him, but then my phone rang. "Hi Philip, it's Len. I've been meaning to call you. The numbness in my extremities that I'd had for two years was gone the very next day after our session. Also, my stress was relieved and my tendonitis is completely gone too! Most importantly, I had another follow up MRI and the malformation has apparently shrunken from the size of a quarter to the size of a dime. The need for surgery has been averted."

The doctors apparently were astonished by the outcome. They said it was impossible.

Over the following year or two, I heard from Len asking for my assistance on a few other matters, including on behalf of a friend who had hurt her right shoulder ten years previously and could find no relief. She called me the very next day after that session. "I don't know what you did, but all the pain is now gone."

EPILEPSY

"I could black out at any time. I'll never drive or ride again."

Christine and I first met in a metaphysical/spiritual bookstore. We had lots in common and we became great friends. She is also into fitness and health, with a thriving home-based business on a ranch north of Toronto. In addition to caring for her animals, one of her greatest passions is driving a Harley Davidson. Recently, she had been experiencing epileptic seizures and was on strong medications to try and keep the unpredictable seizures under control. The prospect of no longer being able to drive or ride was a huge issue for her.

She was open to having some healing sessions, so I went to her ranch. Christine had three sessions, all of which went well. She now has a full and normal life, teaches yoga, and continues to ride her beloved Harley!

BLOCKED SALIVA GLAND

"I can't eat or drink. The pain is unbearable."

It was a bleak Monday evening in early December. The door opened slowly to reveal a tall, elegant young woman. I smiled and introduced myself and her eyes searched my face for a fleeting second, looking for...what? Hope, perhaps? With a wince of pain, she smiled back slightly.

We sat in her living room and, after exchanging pleasantries, she described her medical condition. Judy could not eat and could barely drink. On a pain and discomfort scale she was at a 10 plus. Her sub-mandible saliva gland duct was blocked with a large stone nearly 6mm (¼ inch) in size. The gland had also become infected. A prominent ENT (ear, nose, and throat) specialist had tried unsuccessfully in a two-hour operation to surgically remove the stone. She sought second opinions and all the ENTs had told her that the only medical recourse was to have her entire saliva gland removed. As a doctor herself she knew that a life without a saliva gland would also be intolerable, not to mention that there could also be permanent nerve damage to her face. She simply had to explore another avenue of possibility, no matter how outlandish it might seem, and thus the call to me.

Judy and I continued to speak at length about what was and had been going on in her life, recently and in the more distant past. A discomfort in her neck and jaw had been part of her life for nine years that seemed to worsen during emotional upset and stress. To me there was an obvious connection, but often the person suffering does not see it.

Judy seemed to be open to the possibility of non-physical healing, so after about 45 minutes we began. With some soothing music playing, I spoke quietly to her as she lay on my healing table. Slowly, she drifted away into a sleep-like state while I placed my hands gently on, around, and above her jaw, mouth, and neck. We ended our session and agreed to meet again in two days. I provided her with some positive thoughts and affirmations to focus on before our next session, that would allow the conscious and unconscious mind to do their parts to support the process further.

When we met again Judy's spirits seemed brighter and she was excited to report that the pain she had been experiencing had reduced significantly from a 10 to a more tolerable 4. She was no longer taking any Percocet for the pain.. During our talk, Judy said that her concerns were now more with the blockage and swelling under her tongue and the discharge from the infection. She rated both of these as a 9 out of 10 on the misery scale.

I reminded Judy of the miraculous being she was already and emphasized that in each and every moment her physical body was performing millions and millions of complex functions without any conscious effort on her part. Her Essential Self was taking care of all these functions. I suggested that this is a part of her that is not generally known to the conscious mind, the ego, or intellect. On the table once again, she drifted off into a relaxed sleep-like state while the energies flowed gently and lovingly in and around her being. As we completed, we again agreed to meet in two days time.

On my third visit Judy told me that after our last meeting she had run to the bathroom and had to spit something out. Amazingly, she was also able to eat again! Judy was excited to tell me that the misery index for the swelling under her tongue and the infection was now only at a 2! The pain had gone. There was only a small bubble under her tongue and only a very slight discomfort on the left side of her neck.

I spoke to Judy a few weeks after that session. In the intervening time, she had had new x-rays that came back with the following reading: No calculi. The stone was completely gone!

ACID REFLUX

"For a long time I experienced the constant threat and misery of acid reflux disease."

Roy, a vital and distinguished gentleman, came to me at age 89. He had suffered with acid reflux for a long time, including a dreadful burning in his throat and stomach, and an appalling taste in his mouth. He had to be very careful about what and when he ate and would often be awakened during the night with great pain and discomfort. Roy's medical doctor had prescribed endless amounts of Gaviston pills for the symptoms but offered no actual remedy. The pills did little to relieve the unrelenting pain, discomfort, and burning sensation. The acidic, acrid taste in his mouth continued to be intolerable.

I asked Roy if he would like to have a healing session right there and then, where he stood chatting outside. He readily agreed (although he was concerned about what the neighbors might say!) I stood next to him and put my hand on his solar plexus and on his back. Right away, the energies began and I started to feel the familiar heat. We stood there for about 10 minutes and then we were complete.

The next day Roy reported that he had slept right through the entire night and that the burning feeling and taste was totally gone. In just one 10-minute session the condition completely disappeared!

It has been over a year now and Roy continues to be free of all the former acid reflux pain and discomfort and can pretty well eat whatever he likes.

"I'm overjoyed now to report that after just a few minutes with Philip, my discomfort has all but vanished!! It has truly been a life-changing experience for me. Philip is a miracle worker!"

SHOULDER AND NECK PAIN

"I don't know what you did, but my pain has been completely cured."

Whitney attended a special restorative yoga class of about a dozen people, where I was able to spend about six or seven minutes with each participant in a healing class setting. She reported that, in just those few minutes, I was able to completely heal her long-standing shoulder and neck problems.

KNEE PROBLEMS

"I can hardly walk, I can't skate. All my practice will be wasted."

Mary was a pre-teen figure skater. She had been unable to skate for some time due to a nasty fall. Her parents took her to physical therapists and specialists throughout the Toronto area with no success. Now, her father brought her to me, literally carrying her in. I spoke with Mary as she lay on a couch while her dad sat outside by the window enjoying the afternoon sun. As I spoke to her and put my hands on her knees and legs, she drifted off into a deep relaxation. After about an hour she was complete and said she felt as if she had been on a wonderful vacation and gave a vivid account of all kinds of beautiful colors while in this dream-like state. The next day, her parents were dumbfounded as they watched her perform skating jumps with ease.

Mary said, "After I saw you, I could walk again, and the very next day I was actually doing figure skating jumps for the first time in five months. I am not going to miss the nationals after all. Thank you so much!"

TEETH AND ROOT CANAL

"I have terrible tooth pain. Another root canal will cost me thousands!"

Over the years, Clare had had a number of painful and expensive root canals. Recently, the pain began again and her dentist recommended yet another. Clare had received a number of healing sessions from me for other health and wellness concerns and, when I asked her, said she was open to trying some healing on her jaw and teeth as well.

As she lay back deeply relaxed on her couch, I gently cradled her right jaw and touched her lower molars. After about an hour, we were complete and the next day, the pain had gone. Clare cancelled the root canal procedure with her dentist and is problem-free to this day. In just one session we eliminated the pain and we eliminated the issue.

FOOT PROBLEMS

"I'm afraid my life is over."

Hanna had severe foot problems and was not able to walk properly. Her job of 25 years required her to be mobile and on her feet all day so this issue was completely debilitating. When we met, I spoke to Hanna and explained to her about the strength and power of non-physical energies. I touched her arm and heart. After that the pain in Hanna's feet went away.

Hanna says, "I thought my life was over because I could not walk. If I couldn't walk I would not be able to work. Now I can walk pain-free again. You are my savior! I am so grateful. Thank you!"

CHEST PAIN AND FIBROID TUMORS

"All my life I have been in pain. Now, I feel wonderful."

Kaitlin is a nurse. She had experienced severe and unrelenting pain in her upper chest all her life. There was no known medical cause found, even after every type of medical test had been conducted. She also had dreadful pain in her lower abdomen due to two inoperable fibroid tumors. After her first healing session, the pain in her upper chest left completely. After the second, the intolerable pain in her lower abdomen disappeared.

Kaitlin says, "Now I feel wonderful! Thank you!"

There are, of course, many, many more anecdotes covering almost every imaginable type of malady, but this is all the room we have for now. As the authority on energy healing, I hope that you have found this chapter to be helpful as an introduction to such an expansive metaphysical topic. The concepts may be new to you, although the principles have always been used, in every part of the world, throughout history.

If you feel that I may be able to assist you or a loved one, please call me in Toronto at 416-447-9550. If there is a good fit with us and we do work together, I will visit you in the privacy of your own home and I will commit to working with you until you are completely well again. In the meantime, may blessings of Love and Light always be upon you.

Thank you for your interest! You can learn more at www.PhilipYoungHealer.com

The Get-Back-Up Revolution

Overcome Depression, Failure and Fear in 10 Simple Steps

Jean Kor

Failures, broken relationships, illnesses, deaths of loved ones, injuries, lost moments of greatness, or sometimes just sheer stupidity, occur in our lives at one point or another. We have all had times when we doubt ourselves, when our fear keeps us from daring to follow our heart's desire. There are days when everything seems to go wrong, when we make mistakes and feel like hiding from the world.

There are days, too, when it is even hard to get out of bed, let alone do something that needs to get done. Worse still, when we sit in these feelings for too long, we fall into a downward spiral of despair, hopelessness and depression.

Professional help is always an option but, all too often, that leads to medication. If you are like me, you would much rather find a solution that does not involve prescription drugs or years of therapy. Plus, many of these negative emotions are often based on real life problems that require you to "snap out of it," immediately, and on your own.

Sometimes things that happen to you may seem horrible, unfair and painful at first but, if you take a step back, you will see that it is through these challenging times you are able to find strength, courage, beauty and love in yourself and your surroundings in the most unexpected ways.

Believe me, I know. At one point in my life, I was overwhelmed by fear and despair. I was living as two people. Privately, I was an emotional wreck, fearful, lonely and depressed. I was struggling to save my marriage. My grandma died after a long illness that began with a stroke, and immediately afterwards my mum was diagnosed with cancer. The thought of losing her, my husband and more loved ones further consumed me. I regretted my migration to Canada, and regretted the fact that I did not spend more time with my family.

To make matters worse, my finances suffered, and I misjudged several important decisions. I was broken — I felt like a failure as a daughter, a wife and a leader of my sisters. I hated myself, my life and everything that was happening to me. Publicly, I was the rock on which my family could depend. Quietly, I cried alone for many nights.

THE CHAOS OF MY MIND

I kept telling myself, "All this is beyond my control. There's nothing that I can do. I am so pitiful. I am such a loser." All the while, the dialogue in my head was so negative.

When you keep telling yourself the same story over and over again, you end up believing it. *Instead of finding solutions, I was looking for people and things to blame.* I was stuck in a negative, unproductive place and could not find the light. I isolated myself from my friends and my family, and further spiraled into a deeper state of depression.

Staying in a negative place is unhealthy; not just emotionally, but physically. My health deteriorated. The doctors were puzzled. Multiple tests, heart exams and MRI's later, no major medical problems could be found. It was stress and depression causing all my ailments, and I could feel myself rotting away in despair. I hated how I felt. I wanted my life to improve, but I didn't know how to make the change. In my mind, my problems were insurmountable. They were unsolvable puzzles with no possible solutions.

I craved something more, something better, but just didn't know how to tone down 'the negative voices' I heard constantly and find the positive shift I needed. I didn't know where to start. Then, I realized that I was the only one holding the missing pieces of the jigsaw puzzle I was trying to solve. I was always waiting for a divine intervention, a miracle and someone to help me solve my problems. *Instead of always seeking external advice and approval, what I actually needed was to decide take charge of my life and help myself up to my feet.*

SNAPPING OUT OF IT!

One night, dwelling in self-pity and loneliness, I thought, "I don't want to feel sad tonight; I am just too exhausted for this. I need to snap out of it!" In that instant, I remembered being a kid and playing with an inflatable roly-poly toy filled with sand at the base. I remembered punching it and wrestling it to the ground but, regardless of how hard I tried to keep it down, the toy would always bounce back up to its feet. I thought how nice it would be if I had one of those with me at the moment.

That night, I had a purpose. I decided to make one of those toys to cheer myself up. Immediately, my focus changed, and I forgot about my problems. I started looking for ways to make the toy. I took out my sewing machine, cut up an old t-shirt, took stuffing from a pillow, and made myself a roly-poly bunny — truth be told, a pretty crummy looking bunny filled with rice at the base. But ...It was soft and comforting. I pushed it down, and it immediately got back up to its feet, and that put a big smile on my face. It was exactly as I remembered.

Then I drew a zany expression with squinty eyes on the blank bunny face. I wanted the face to represent life's journey. The squiggly mouth I drew meant that life was full of ups and downs. The fact that the smile ended in an upturn meant that, despite all the challenges, life would end with an upward victory smile!

"Stay strong, bunny! Get back on your feet and never give up!" I spoke out loud to the bunny, but it wasn't the bunny that needed to hear those words. I needed the positive words of encouragement.

Now, the crummy looking bunny I made wasn't invincible. After several falls, it got stuck in an awkward position and couldn't get back up to its feet. However, when I gave it a little nudge, it quickly bounced back up again. It reminded me of the many times when I had hard times, made mistakes or felt like a failure and my family and friends were always there to love me unconditionally, and help me up to my feet again.

When I looked at my bunny, I saw *perseverance, strength, positivity, gratitude, love* and *support*. It felt alive and real. I was so excited by my discovery that the resilient bunny I had created could help me feel so much better so quickly. He could be knocked down, but he always got back up, just like what I needed to do.

I quickly shot a video of my bunny and immediately shared it with my family and friends. They all loved it! Everyone wanted one as it resonated with the daily struggles they all had in lives. It soon got the nickname the *NEVER GIVE UP BUNNY* because of the symbolic message of resiliency it demonstrates.

A DECISION TO SHIFT MY FOCUS

I knew then that I couldn't change the things that had happened, but I could change how I felt in any given moment. | wanted to be happy. I wanted to have a happy relationship. I wanted to be fit and healthy again. I wanted to make my parents happy. I wanted to be successful. I wanted to be someone that my siblings looked up to. I wanted to be able to cheer my family up and improve their lives.

I knew I must make a change in order to be happy. I resolved to change my attitude first. By shifting to positive questions, focusing on what I wanted (and not what I hated), *I started to find solutions to get the results I craved.* Before, my problems were huge, unsolvable puzzles. Now I know that I don't need to wait for all the answers to overcome my problems. Instead of being overwhelmed, I can just start by taking it one tiny step at a time. By breaking down a problem into a series of small achievable tasks, I can then easily tackle each task until I achieve all the goals I have set. That shift in approaching a problem would change how I felt about finding a solution.

HELPING OTHERS

I had wanted my family and friends to have the same feeling of comfort and confidence that I had found in my zany *NEVER GIVE UP BUNNY*. During my darkest moments, my bunny helped me find the courage to pick myself up, dust myself off and get 'hopping' once again.

So, over the next few months I looked back at my struggles and journey and came up with a ten step plan for overcoming depression, failure, lack of motivation, fear and self-doubt. These steps will help propel you into a world where answers can be found in difficult situations and trying times.

Step 1: Get Serious and Decide — Do You Want Things to Change?

If you don't like your current situation, then decide that you really want it to change and *get serious* about it! Only you have the power to make that decision. *"For things to change, first you have to change."* Change sounds scary, but, if you want new results you have to be willing to give it a go. If you keep doing what you've been doing, you'll keep on getting what you have been getting. I understand that most of us are fearful of change because of the uncertainties that lie ahead. Don't be scared!

Step 2: Take a Timeout – Stop Complaining and Be Thankful

Stop the negative inner dialogue. Don't be preoccupied with hating everything around you, complaining about everything and thinking that everything is going against you. You need room to see, feel, realize and receive the good things happening around you. Some of us would find ways to 'dis' every good thing and make believe that it was, indeed, a negative. When you focus on what you hate or dislike, that is exactly what you are going to find. *Remember that you are only as pathetic as you believe yourself to be.*

Emotional hurts don't last unless you hang on to them. Don't let harsh words linger in your mind creating a negative dialogue that gets bigger as you repeat it and dwell in it.

Be thankful. Take a moment to stop and think about all the good things that have happened to you. As dire as things may seem at the moment, dig deep and find the littlest thing that you can be thankful for. I created a gratitude journal. I started with being thankful for a blessed life, an able body, having a roof above my head, food on the table, great friends and family who loves me. Then I started seeing beauty in the little things I took for granted, and I became thankful for the smiling cashier, a chat with friends over coffee, the smooth traffic and the extra nut I found on my banana nut muffin.

Step 3: Tell Yourself You Deserve to Be Happy

Eventually, your inner dialogue will change. You will understand that you are valuable and deserve all the positive changes happening in your life. God made everyone equal and does not discriminate. Regardless of whom you are, what your background is, or what your past was, the only thing that matters is the present and what we do to create a better tomorrow.

Oprah Winfrey said, "Change is possible. Greatness is possible. But you can't do anything unless you first believe in yourself." So, hold your head up high because you have every right to do so. Tell yourself you are a special person and a great individual. Believe in yourself, because if you don't, no one else will. Start by writing down 50-100 reasons why you deserve all the good things in life and why you love yourself. Include your strengths, skills and good qualities. You do not have to be shy or humble in this exercise. Go ahead — compliment, praise and love yourself for any reason.

Step 4: Take Responsibility for Your Own Life

It is easier to find excuses, dodge the issues and always put the blame on others. By doing so, we leave our lives in other people's hands — always playing the helpless victim, waiting and hoping for help that may never come. In order to take charge of our lives and destiny, we need to be self-reliant and understand that nobody owes us anything. You have to be responsible for your own needs, emotions, physical well-being, economic, social or spiritual. Stop figuring out why and how you fell into the hole you are in. Instead, start thinking about how to get out. Stop waiting for help. Help yourself. You have to take action.

Step 5: Set Your Goals, Be Clear About What You Want

Clarity is power. The clearer the reason for change, the easier it will be to accomplish your goal. Ask yourself: "Why do I want to change?" Associate the end goal with all the pleasure and possible delightful results. Consider all the pain, suffering and negative consequences of staying where you. Let these immense visualizations be your driving force. You need to understand, change is never a matter of ability. It is a matter of motivation, of having the desire to create that change.

Set your goals; break them down into simple, small and achievable tasks. Work on a plan to become more organized and tackle the tasks you have been avoiding. Having a goal to work on gives you a sense of purpose and, just by working on it, you will immediately feel happier.

Step 6: Get the Tools and Take Action

Knowing what you want to change and why you want to change it is just the first step in creating positive change. *You have to take action. Not just small action but MASSIVE, EARTH SHATTERING ACTION!* Equip yourself with the right "tools' to achieve your goals and attain the results that you want.

144

Go back to school, get a treadmill, get more training and invest in yourself. If you find that the tool you have is not producing the results you want, switch it up, get a different tool and make it happen.

Step 7: Change Your Inner Dialogue

You have the goals, you understand the reasons, and you have the tools. Why have you not followed through? You may have hit a small obstacle. Your inner demon may be talking to you. It's saying, "I knew this would not work." You believe it because that is the conversation you have had with yourself for years. *Stop it!* You can do this. Change your perspective and tackle that obstacle. Instead of focusing on the problem, focus on the solutions. If you keep telling yourself that change is good and that you can do it, eventually you will believe it.

Step 8: Conquer your Fear

Everybody is afraid. Have you ever ridden a rollercoaster? The reason why it is so exciting is because you are testing the limits of what is safe. People who design roller coasters have found a way to use fear and turn it into a thrilling experience. You need to find a *way to use your fear to propel you into action* instead of letting it destroy you. Don't pretend that fear is not there. Challenge yourself. If you are afraid, ask yourself, "Will a negative result be worse than doing nothing and maintaining the status quo?" Focus on what you want, not what you are afraid of. Change your inner dialogue.

Step 9: Anticipate Challenges & Reward Yourself

Life is not a straight path. Anticipate that there will be ups and downs along the way, and don't be overly stressed up when you hit a bump on the road. There are many forks in the road. Look at the possible outcomes and evaluate them. There will be challenges and road blocks, and you might even make the wrong turn occasionally, but that is as anticipated. Admit it. Then change it. Every wrong turn brings you closer to your end destination as long as you keep on going and don't give up. In knowing this, you will be calm in the face of adversity. Remember to celebrate and reward yourself for your actions and successes. You are your greatest critic or your loudest cheerleader. Be a cheerleader!

Step 10: Create and Maintain a Strong Positive Foundation

For anything to grow, it must have a strong foundation and a robust environment. Create and cultivate a group of people who love and support you. Find people who challenge you to be better, and encourage you to try new solutions. Find workshops that add new tools to your toolkit. Keep expanding your expectations. Last but not least, taking care of the health of our minds and bodies is fundamental for ensuring that we will have the energy and vitality to create the life we want. For me, the moment I decided to take responsibility for my own life and not let depression consume me, I felt powerful, alive and free from the shackles in which I had bound myself. Having long-term goals to work on gives me a purpose and helps me grow each day. I have started a blog sharing fun and inspirational materials as well as the zany looking bunny which was, and still is, my source of strength and a constant reminder of perseverance.

It has not been smooth sailing. Trust me, there were many, many times when I struggled hard and just wanted to give up. It certainly was not easy, but I am glad that I found the strength to get back up to my feet and make a positive difference in this world.

You may never know exactly what tomorrow holds for you, but for now, smile through your tears, laugh at the confusion, wink at the fear, and remind yourself to stay strong always. Never ever give up. Pick yourself up, create the life you deserve and live life with absolutely no regrets.

If you know someone who could use a *NEVER GIVE UP BUNNY* or want to share your personal journey with me, please visit www.nevergiveupbunny. com.

Family Is Everything

DAN ROGERS

Hundreds of years ago wooden ships brought immigrants to the shores of what would become the maritime provinces of Canada. Why did the pioneers brave starvation, malnutrition, disease or shipwreck?

Today, a number of immigrants arrived at Pearson International Airport in Toronto, Ontario. Why did they leave their countries, their jobs and friends to try and carve out a new life in Canada?

Ask such questions of either group and you would likely receive the identical answer: "To build a better life for my family," they would say. Why? Because family is everything!

In 1916 a young couple, Clarence and Lizzy, got married and boarded a train to northwest Saskatchewan. The rules were that if you were over eighteen, married and agreed to live on and work the land, the government would grant you a quarter section, which is 160 acres or 65 hectares.

At first they plowed the virgin fields with a team of oxen. The prairie grass roots were so thick that the girl had to follow along behind the plow, cutting the roots of the prairie grass with a butcher knife. Her first three babies miscarried. Then, on her fourth pregnancy, the boy rounded up just enough money for one train ticket to the closest town that had a hospital (Lloydminster). He took her in a horse drawn wagon across the prairie for many kilometers to the train station, put her on the train and returned home to continue working the fields. The girl gave birth to a healthy baby girl named Grace. That baby girl was my mother.

My grandmother was what was known as a Bernardo child. She was in a program based out of England that was founded by a man named Bernardo. Orphans and children whose parents could not afford to look after them were shipped to Canada to live on farms. Some of the families treated the child as one of their own, while others treated the child as a slave. The end result, however, was that they got to Canada. And it worked, albeit slowly. So ... my mother had a better life than her mother ... I am having a better life than my mother ... and my son, an only child, came home from the hospital not only to his own bedroom, but to one that had a four piece en suite bathroom. Also, by the time my wife and I are gone from this world, he will be an automatic millionaire.

My hope is that you and your family can accomplish this quicker than we did. We were slow learners. It took us over a century to create wealth. But the fact that you are in Canada and reading this book already puts you in the group that is most likely to succeed. Do you find that hard to believe? Then just think of all the people who came home from work today and are either checking Facebook or watching reality TV. They definitely aren't reading a book about how to succeed financially.

THE PURPOSE OF THIS CHAPTER

The purpose of this chapter is to help educate you to use whatever money you have to benefit you and your family in the long run.

The first thing I want to do is ask you a question: What is your biggest asset? Many people will answer that question by stating what they own. Various answers will be the most obvious ones like my house, my car, my life insurance policy, my retirement fund. But the real answer is you or, to be more accurate, it's your ability to earn a living.

Now, consider that the average annual income in Canada is around fifty thousand dollars (at time of printing). That means in a typical forty year career you will have grossed two million dollars. Yet, most Canadians don't own two million dollars of mortgage free real estate or don't have two million dollars in the bank or even in an insurance policy. Why is that?

It's simple mathematics …

Mr. A and Mr. B both moved to Canada about fifty years ago from the same country. They both got jobs at the same company for the same wage. But Mr. A saved up his money for a down payment on a house and also budgeted in the monthly premium for a permanent life insurance policy, while Mr. B spent much of his disposable income on trips back to his homeland, coffee shops, take- out food, and cigarettes.

Both A and B died about twenty years ago. The daughter of Mr. A inherited a mortgage free house and a life insurance policy, while the son of Mr. B ended up with nothing. Because the child of A immediately had cash in hand, from the insurance money, and she chose to live in the house for free, she was able to invest both the life insurance money and the monthly rent she had previously been paying. Meanwhile, the son of Mr. B had to save for years and years before he could get out of the apartment he was renting, because saving up while paying rent is much more challenging. In the end, however, B descendent was able to buy a house and make some modest investments.

Eventually the heirs of both Mr. A and Mr. B died. The grandchildren of A have inherited multiple real estate properties and investment funds easily worth in excess of a million dollars, while the family of Mr. B ended up with only a few hundred thousand, as the real estate and other investments were purchased later in their parents' lives and didn't have time enough to grow. The property may not have even been mortgage free at the time of Mr. B's death.

So, the third generation of the A family are now millionaires, while the same generation of the B family has enough money for a modest down payment on a nice house.

You want to be Mr or Mrs A. Buy a home early and pay off that mortgage. Protect your ability to earn with the proper insurance policies and invest on an ongoing basis. Read on, I'll show you how to do it. But first a discussion about estate planning

WILL AND POWER OF ATTORNEY

We have been talking about estates. These are passed on to beneficiaries through the vehicle known as the will. But, over the several years that I have been in this profession, I have encountered a rather high percentage of people that do not have their wills done. And you do need one. Not a "do it yourself" will kit that can be purchased online or at a business supply retailer. Generally, the legal system does not consider this type of will to be valid. No, I strongly urge you to have a lawyer draw up your will. A good lawyer. A conscientious lawyer. Here's why …

An elderly widower sells his house, puts the money in the bank, moves to an apartment, and marries a much younger new wife. His lawyer draws up a will stating that his estate will be divided amongst his wife, his three children and his two favourite charities. The lawyer did not enquire about what type of account the money was in or ask any questions of that nature. When the man died, the executor of the estate found out that the bank had advised the man to name a beneficiary to the account, so the man, not being given a full legal explanation of the ramifications, named his wife as beneficiary. So, on his death, the bank immediately transferred 100% of the funds into the wife's name, and there was no legal recourse to get her to divide up the money according to the will. The will became a useless piece of paper. The three children and the two charities received nothing from the fund. That man was my father.

The lesson to be learned is to never assume that a professional you hire is automatically going to do things in your best interest.

Power of Attorney: There are two types of power of attorney: one for personal care, and one for property. This means that you designate a person to make decisions on your behalf should you reach the point where you can no longer make these decisions yourself. **Personal care** refers to topics such as choosing a personal support worker, a nursing home, treatments, medications, and other things of that nature. **Property** refers to topics such as whether or not to sell the house or rent it out or authorize repairs, and whether to sell the car, or cut the lawn or many other property related items.

In listing a power of attorney, remember that you do not have to have the same person for all areas. You could have a daughter who would be the best for personal care, an eldest son who would make the best executor, and a youngest son who is in real estate who would be the best person for property decisions.

I should also mention **Probate** as it is a complicated and frequently costly procedure wherein you must prove the validity of the will. The general rule is that if there is a beneficiary listed on the account, then probate is not required.

When the funds are in a bank, the money could be in one of several different types of accounts. It could be in a chequing account, a savings account, a TFSA (tax free savings account), an RRSP (registered retirement savings plan), mutual funds, segregated funds, GIC (guaranteed investment certificate), a RIF (retirement income fund), and a number of others. The bank would likely ask you to name a beneficiary on the account. This is done to prevent probate. However, remember the story about my father and learn from it. If there is only one person that you want to give your money to, then that is fine, but if there are multiple people, you must name them all.

PROTECT YOURSELF

In order to open this discussion, we need to go back to the reason everyone comes to Canada in the first place. We all know the answer to that one: to build a better life for your family. At the same time, we need to recall your greatest asset. It's you, and if you go down, everything that you worked for could be lost. So we are going to address a very important issue, income replacement. This is generally broken down into two areas; disability coverage and critical illness coverage.

Disability coverage: Disability insurance is meant to replace part of your income (usually 55%) in case of injury or illness. Now, the first thing to know is that not all disability policies are equal. Some give you the right see your own doctor—some do not. And that makes all the difference. The first group of claimants tends to be entrepreneurs who don't want to be away from their jobs any longer than the insurance company wants them to be. The second group of claimants tends to be more the corporate type, a type that encompasses malingerers—those people who are in no rush to get back to work after an injury or illness—the type that breeds distrust in the insurance companies. Make sure you're in the first group.

Integration of benefits: What this means is that if you signed up for a $2,000/month disability policy and you get hurt, and another organization also agrees to pay you let's say $1,200/month, whether it is another insurance company, Workers Safety Insurance Board, the employer, or whomever, then your insurance company only has to pay you the difference of $800/month. You can find policies that don't have this clause.

Return of Premium: What if you are lucky and never get injured? How would you like to get all your money back when you retire, tax free? Yes, there are disability policies available that have this benefit.

Soft tissue injuries/back injuries/sprains/strains: This is another very important feature. Many disability providers are so concerned about people faking injuries that they won't pay out unless something shows up on an X-ray. You don't want a policy like that. You want a policy that will cover you in all cases of injury or illness.

Injury occurs on or off the job: Many employers who provide a benefit plan to their employees will have disability coverage that only covers on the job accidents. While better than nothing, statistically, the average Canadian is more likely to get hurt in a car accident, at home, or while participating in sports and leisure than actually getting hurt on the job. That' the kind of coverage you want.

No limit on number of claims made: This one is fairly self-explanatory.

Make sure your provider does not have a clause where they can terminate your coverage if you make too many claims.

Critical Illness/Hospital Sickness Benefits: Let's imagine that you or your spouse were diagnosed with a terminal illness or a debilitating disease. The ill person might wish to do their "bucket list," go back to visit the homeland, see the Seven Wonders of the World, or take a cruise around the world. But from where would the money come? Cash in RRSPs? Sell the house? Remortgage the house? The problem with doing that is it ruins the whole game plan of coming to Canada to build a better life for your children and your children's children.

This is the reason that critical illness coverage exists in a place that already has state funded health care.

And just like disability coverage, it is possible to get critical illness coverage with a Return of Premium Clause, meaning that if you remain in good health, you get your money back at the end.

LIFE INSURANCE

There are many different types of life insurance. It is vitally important for you to know the differences so that you can pick the type that is the right one for your situation.

Reason for life insurance: Do you have massive debt from a mortgage or business loan that if all goes well you will have paid off before retirement? Or do you want to leave your family a lump sum of money for a particular purpose, regardless of whether you die young or old? These two situations require (differing) insurance products.

The standard formula that the insurance industry uses for determining the amount of coverage is: ten times annual salary plus debt. So if you make the average Canadian income of about $50,000 per year and have a three hundred thousand dollar mortgage, then the calculation would be to have $800,000 in coverage.

Term Insurance: Term insurance would be better understood by the public if it were renamed "temporary insurance." With term insurance you are buying a window of time. If you die in that window of time, the insurance company writes a cheque to your beneficiary. If you die outside that window, they cut no cheque at all.

Permanent insurance: Permanent insurance is frequently known by its official name, whole life insurance. If the reason for buying is that you need some security to pay off your debts if you die young, then term is the way to go, but if you want to leave a lump sum to your family whether you die next year or in sixty years, then you will want a permanent product.

Term to 100: Term to 100 is a rather unique type of life insurance that is sort of a hybrid between term insurance and permanent insurance. As we have already read, the disadvantage of a term policy is that it eventually runs out, but the advantage is lower premiums. The disadvantage of whole life coverage is that the premiums are high, but the advantage is that it lasts forever. What if you could get a policy that never runs out but that has the lower premiums more associated with term insurance? Great, right? That's why many companies don't offer the product. But you can find it, if that is what you want.

No Medical Insurance: No medical insurance is frequently called other names such as final expense insurance, funeral insurance, burial insurance, guaranteed issue insurance, instant issue insurance, and perhaps a few other names. It is frequently advertised by way of television commercials, and mail flyers delivered by the post office. The target client is often a retiree whose term insurance has now expired but who still wants to leave a lump sum when he or she dies. People with health problems who will never qualify for standard application coverage also tend to buy this type of policy.

Universal Life: This is another type of whole life policy. It can be a bit complicated, so I'm going to give a brief explanation of this product here. With a universal life policy, a portion of your premium goes into an investment. Over the years, the idea is for the investment to grow substantially. A universal life policy with a face amount of $100,000 would have an additional investment portion attached to it, so after a few decades the policy might pay out in total $150,000, $200,000 or more. Although this seems like a great idea, low interest rates over the past several years have made many people who hold a universal life policy realize that the projected payout at the end is going to be considerably lower than what the agent had suggested way back when the policy was first taken out.

The moral of this story is to make sure you sit down with a financial professional who will do a "needs analysis."

PLANNING FOR RETIREMENT

RRSP stands for Registered Retirement Savings Plan. An RRSP isn't an investment, it's a shell in which you can store all sorts of different kinds of financial plans and investments.

An RRSP could contain stocks, bonds, mutual funds, segregated funds, Guaranteed Investment Certificates, syndicate mortgages, Guaranteed Investment Accounts, just to name some of the more popular products that a typical Canadian RRSP might contain.

What an RRSP does is let you defer income tax. It is designed for Canadians who know that they are going to be bringing in less money after they retire than they are currently bringing in now. Canada Revenue Agency (CRA) charges income tax on a sliding scale depending on the income of the person. Someone who doesn't earn much income may pay no income tax at all, where someone with a high income might pay out 40% of their pay to income tax.

Life Income Fund: A life income fund generally comes from a company pension. Some employers offer a company matched retirement plan, meaning that whatever you put into it, they will contribute an equal amount. When you leave the company, it is recommended that you do something with it. The reason is that if the company runs into financial trouble, your retirement fund could be gone, or at least reduced. It has happened before, and will most likely happen again. Instead, if you quit, get downsized, or retire, you should move that money out of there and put it with an investment firm. That way, the success of your former employer will have no influence on the fund.

Various investments

Mutual funds are what are known as securities. The agent or broker must hold a license regulated by each provinces securities commission. Mutual funds are really just a collection of various stocks. They were designed for the purpose of the small investor being able to get into the stock market without a large cash outlay and with a lower risk. There are thousands of different funds out there, and virtually all of them are quite heavily diversified. This is both good news and bad news. The good news is that if one or a few of the companies that are inside that particular mutual fund take a huge nose dive, it won't cause your fund to drop too dramatically. The bad news is really the opposite side of the same coin. If a few of the stocks in the fund soar tremendously, your fund won't go up all that much because of all the other stocks in there that remain steadfast or have dropped. Mutual funds have no guarantees whatsoever, so if your fund dropped way down, you have only two choices: you can cash out at a loss, or you can hold onto it for enough years and hope that it rebounds satisfactorily. Mutual funds are also subject to fees known as Management Expense Ratios, or MER. If your fund's MER is 2%, then on a one hundred thousand dollar investment, expect to pay two thousand dollars per year in fees.

Segregated funds are very similar in concept to mutual funds. Segregated funds are sold by life insurance companies. Many financial experts describe segregated funds as "mutual funds with an insurance policy wrapper". Segregated funds must be kept separate from the insurance company's regular finances, hence the name. A "seg" fund and a mutual fund may both be investing in the same stocks, the main difference between the two, is there is a guarantee with a seg fund. The guarantee in a seg fund is generally either 75% or 100% of the original investment, depending on which plan you take. That means that you are guaranteed to get back either 75% or 100% of your money, even if the fund loses money. You will have to hold onto the fund for an agreed upon length of time, usually ten years to get this guarantee. And it is important to know that this guarantee is not free. A seg fund will have extra fees associated with it to cover this guarantee. If you cash out before the agreed upon time, you get what is in the fund, whether it has gained money or lost money, less any fees. If the seg fund rises in value, most plans will allow you to "reset" the guaranteed amount to this higher amount, however, that would mean that doing this will reset the amount of time, usually ten years, that you must hold the fund.

Depending on which plan you take, 75% or 100%, if you die while the funds are down, your beneficiary will receive 75% or 100% of the fund.

Guaranteed Investment Certificate (GIC): A GIC is a savings account where the interest rate is pre-set. There is an amount of time, generally two years, three years, four years, or five years that you must keep the money in the account in order to obtain that interest rate. If you withdraw the funds earlier than that date, you won't get the agreed upon interest rate. The longer you keep the money locked up, the higher the interest rate you can get.

Guaranteed Investment Account (GIA): The simplest way to describe a GIA is that it is like a GIC, except it is carried by insurance companies, just like seg funds, and the guarantee activates in the event of the contract holder's death.

If the contract holder dies while having a GIA, the company guarantees the highest of the two following things: either the balance of the account on the date of death; or 100% of the sum invested in this account.

Syndicated Mortgages: A developer who wants to build a condo tower, a commercial office building, or any other large construction project can generally only get conventional bank financing up to a certain percentage of the cost of the project. The remainder of the amount he needs has to come from someplace else. When you agree to give the developer your money, you go on title, the same way that your bank is on title for your house, if you have a mortgage. Syndicated mortgages have been around for a long time, but ordinary folk like you and me have only started hearing about them in the past few years. The reason is that they used to be reserved for those with very large sums to invest, like a million dollars. It was only relatively recently that the industry opened up the market dramatically by lowering the minimum investment to twenty five thousand dollars. Generally, the syndicate mortgages that have come across my desk pay 8% per annum, simple interest. It is important to know the difference between simple interest and compound interest. With compound interest, you receive interest on your interest, but with simple interest you do not. A typical syndicate mortgage locks your money away for a period of time, frequently three or four years.

Gold and other precious metals: The only reason that I am even mentioning this topic is because I am told that there are people on the radio urging us to buy gold. On the financial security pyramid or pillars, or ladder, or however you would like to refer to it, precious metals are to be considered at the top, right up there with collecting works of art. This means that it is something that would be recommended to do after your house is mortgage free, and you have amassed considerable wealth and assets.

REAL ESTATE

Buy vs Rent: There are always those who debate whether or not it is better to rent and invest more in the market, or buy real estate, and subsequently have less money left over at the end of the month to invest. Remember that home ownership has two entirely separate goals. The first one is to make money on it, either by buying low and selling high, or by making improvements to the property, thus increasing its value, or by paying off the mortgage so that you no longer have the expense of making payments. The second goal is to improve your quality of life. You have your very own residence without being at the mercy of a landlord, should they decide to sell the property, or raise the rent, or move into it themselves, or move a relative into it. You also have total control over what colour you would like the walls painted, the types of light fixtures, window coverings, faucets, countertops, and a host of other features.

Buying Real Estate: The first thing you will require is the **minimum down payment**. When you buy with less than twenty percent down, this is what the banks refer to as a high ratio mortgage. This requires you to have mortgage default insurance. The most popular organization the banks use to obtain mortgage default insurance is the Canada Mortgage and Housing Corporation (CMHC), a crown corporation. Two other companies that offer this are Genworth Financial Canada, and Canada Guaranty. They will charge a fee, and blend it into your payment. This can only be avoided by having a minimum of twenty percent of the purchase price of the property already saved up and available. For a first time home buyer, this could be difficult. Most of the property purchases I have made had CMHC on them. I still found this to be the lesser of the evils when compared to paying rent.

Next, you will need to **obtain approval for the mortgage**. You should do this before looking at any properties. There are two ways of doing this. The first is to talk to your own bank branch. The second is to use a mortgage broker. The advantage of using a mortgage broker is twofold. First, they do all the work, don't charge you and get paid a referral fee from the financial institution where the mortgage is placed. The second advantage is that they will frequently work with multiple lenders, giving them and you more choices. One thing they will be looking for is your Total Debt Service Ratio (TDSR). This means that all your payments, mortgage, utilities, and other things such as car loan payments and line of credit payments should not exceed approximately forty percent of your overall gross household income. So first of all, you should not be considering real estate if you owe any money on anything else, and yes, that includes your car.

The next thing is your need to have established a **credit rating**. There are two credit rating services. The most popular one is Equifax, and the other one is TransUnion. You can obtain your credit score from these institutions yourself at no charge. They will probably try to get you to pay for it, and they will quite likely offer you the information instantly if you pay, but you can wait and get it the slow way without having to pay. If you are new to the country, or young, or both, you may not have established a credit rating. The first thing is to have a credit card. Obviously, the intended goal is to pay the balance off every statement, thus avoiding any interest payments. If you think you can get by in this world without a credit card, you thought wrong. Not only is it vital in establishing a credit rating, but without one, it is generally quite difficult to purchase anything online, obtain tickets for a major event, rent a car, book a flight, stay in a hotel, and a host of various other situations that will cross your path from time to time.

Types of properties: There are really only four: condo, townhouse, semi, and detached

Condo is short for condominium. You will usually see them in the form of high rise buildings, but there are townhouse condos and even detached condos. With a condo you only own the inside, the condo corporation owns the outside. I'm using simple terminology here. You pay a monthly fee to them and they are responsible for exterior things like the roof, landscaping, snow removal, elevators, and really everything this is not inside your unit.

The next type of property on the scale is the **townhouse**. They can be condos or freehold. If it is a townhouse condo, you pay a fee to the condo corporation, just like a high rise, and they look after the same things like the roof, snow removal, and grass cutting. If it is a freehold, you own the whole thing, and you are responsible for everything. The main items to think about with a townhouse is that you share your walls with someone else.

Next on the list is the **semi-detached**. This has all the same possible downsides as a townhouse, but you are only sharing one wall. The key to a good semi is to have a great neighbour on the other side of the wall. But of course, you have very little way of finding that out until you are already moved in.

A **detached house**, meaning that it is not connected to any other building (you can walk all the way around all four sides), is the ultimate goal, in my humble opinion. In many regions, especially in the Greater Toronto Area (GTA), the detached house is sought after not only for the buffer zone between neighbours, but because many of these houses are ideally suited to having a separate basement apartment with a separate entrance, frequently a side door. This is an excellent way to bring in extra money to offset the high mortgage payment.

GOVERNMENT RETIREMENT BENEFITS

There are five main areas about which you will need to know: Canada Pension Plan (CPP), Canada Pension Plan Survivor Benefit, Canada Pension Plan Death Benefit, Old Age Security (OAS) and Guaranteed Income Supplement (GIS).

The Canada Pension Plan (CPP) is something that you would have paid into during the course of your working career. You can apply for it as early as age sixty or as late as age seventy. If you apply for it at age sixty, you will, however, receive a 36% reduction in benefits. If you apply for it at age seventy, you will get an increase of 42%.

According to the government of Canada statistics as of the year 2015, the average CPP monthly benefit is $619 and the maximum is $1,065.

Old Age Security: The Old Age Security (OAS) is a benefit for which you can apply at age sixty five, as of now, however, there are plans to increase the age at which you can apply to age sixty seven. Time will tell if the federal government sticks to the plan of age sixty seven, or if successive governments decide to roll it back to age sixty five. At time of publishing, the OAS is around $565 per month, however, it is indexed to inflation, so it generally goes up a few dollars per month every year.

CPP Survivor Benefit: If you are the first to die in a spousal or common-law relationship, the surviving spouse should apply for this benefit. It is generally 60% of the deceased partner's monthly CPP benefit, or if death occurs before age sixty five, then this benefit is calculated on the amount that it would have been if death had occurred at age sixty five.

CPP Death Benefit: Only a very few countries offer this benefit. To be eligible for your estate to receive this benefit you must have made contributions to CPP in the lesser of: one third of the calendar years in your CPP contributory period, but no less than three calendar years; or ten calendar years.

The amount of the death benefit depends on how much and for how long the deceased contributed to the CPP. The maximum benefit is $2,500. According to the latest statistics, the average benefit is around $2,300. The CPP death benefit is calculated as the amount equal to six months' worth of your monthly CPP benefit.

Guaranteed Income Supplement (GIS): If you live in Canada and have a low income, this monthly non-taxable benefit can be added to your Old Age Security (OAS) pension, if your annual income (or in case of a couple, your combined income) is less than the maximum annual income. The Canadian government calculates this maximum annual income amount based on numerous different criteria such as if you are single, widowed, or divorced, or if you have a spouse that receives the full OAS pension, or if your spouse does not receive the OAS, or if your spouse is already receiving the GIS and the OAS. You can always go the government's website yourself when you need this information: www.servicecanada.gc.ca

FINAL ARRANGEMENTS

This section will be dealing with an area that most people are not particularly thrilled about discussing. Furthermore, most people are not willing to walk into a funeral home and ask questions. Fortunately, I worked in the industry for ten years, so I'm in the position to not only help you spare your family a lot of grief and hardship, but at the same time, save you money as well.

There are two ways to pre-arrange your funeral: One way is to pre-arrange but not pre-pay. The other, and more preferred way, is to pre-arrange and pre-pay.

Cremation verses Burial: The main reason that 90 % of the people I have talked to about funerals over the years choose cremation, is so they can avoid the cemetery completely.

If you choose cremation, there are five options open to you regarding the disposition of the remains.

1. Your family can take the urn home with them and put it on the shelf. (This is not for everyone, some like the idea, some hate it.)

2. You can have the ashes scattered. Note: this choice is completely legal.

3. If you have an immediate family member that is already in a cemetery plot, most cemetery boards will allow you to place your urn in your family member's plot, generally for a fee of a few hundred dollars.

4. You can purchase your very own plot and have your urn buried there.

5. Cemeteries have structures called columbariums, or wall niches, that you can purchase for the purpose of having your urn placed there permanently.

Funeral Service Choices: For the sake of simplicity, there are really only three.

1. **A Direct Disposition.** All this means is that you are hiring the services of a licensed funeral director to send a transfer vehicle to your place of death, whether that is a hospital, a nursing home, or your own home. They will pick up the remains and transport them back to the preparation room at the funeral home, arrange for the cremation and return the ashes to you.

2. **A Memorial Service** contains everything a direct disposition contains, but the funeral establishment puts on a service, either in their own building, or in the church of your choice. Sometimes people want it to be held in a different location, such as a club that has their own facilities. It is important to note that with a memorial service, the body is not present, no casket is present, cremation has already taken place, and most often, the urn is present in lieu of a casket.

3. **A Traditional Service**: This is the type of arrangement where the casket is present. I'm not sure why, but many people are under the misconception that a traditional service is not available with cremation. The facts are that there are only two real differences between a traditional service with cremation to follow, and a traditional service with burial to follow. The first difference is that with burial, there is a funeral procession from the funeral home or church to the cemetery, and with cremation to follow, there is not, because the body has to be transported to the crematorium. The second difference is that with burial, a casket

is purchased, and the casket is buried. But with cremation, the funeral home usually provides the use of the casket for the visitation and service, and hidden inside the casket underneath the white satin lining, where no one can see, is the combustible, rigid, leak-proof container that is always necessary with cremation.

"I'm donating my body to science!"

This is what you need to know with regards to whole body donation. Medical schools, or schools of anatomy will accept body donations to train future medical professionals. It is completely different than donating organs. The body must be in very good condition and there must be a need for the body. It is important to remember that if you have a pre-paid funeral and you are accepted by a medical school, the pre-paid funeral fund will be returned to the family with interest.

SUMMARY

What do all of these things I've been talking about have in common? The greatest point of all that I've written here is that there are many ways for you to achieve wealth and grow it. An early mortgage and long-term investments can result in a free home for your loved ones to live in, money for them to live on and funds to grow even more money. They can even take the money they used to pay rent with and purchase yet more investments, so that when the third generation matures, there is a literal fortune waiting for them to inherit.

We also discussed investment vehicles such as real estate, mutual funds and term deposits, touching on various types of each, the idea being to make you aware of the choices you have moving forward. We even talked about how to protect your earning potential with disability insurance and life insurance. The chapter ended with a looked at funeral planning.

You came to Canada to make a better life for your family. This chapter can set you on the proper path to achieve what you wish. Good luck in all you do!